D0604624

Men'sHealth®

TOTAL
FITNESS
GUIDE
2008

MUSCLE
CHOW®

≫ MORE THAN 150 EASY-TO-FOLLOW RECIPES
TO BURN FAT AND FEED YOUR MUSCLES

GREGG AVEDON, CPT

RODALE

Photographs by Mitch Mandel/Rodale Images

Book design by Joanna Williams

ISBN-13 978–1–59486–873–3 hardcover
ISBN-10 1–59486–873–5 hardcover

2 4 6 8 10 9 7 5 3 1 hardcover

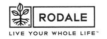

LIVE YOUR WHOLE LIFE

We inspire and enable people to improve their lives and the world around them

For more of our products visit **rodalestore.com** or call 800-848-4735

CONTENTS

CONTENTS

FOREWORD

Gregg Avedon and I have a lot in common. Okay, maybe I don't have his physique (not even close), but the fact that I haven't appeared on any *Men's Health* covers doesn't sever the bonds that tie us together. We both love food, are fascinated by the field of nutrition, and have the dubious challenge of managing busy careers while striving to spend more time with the beautiful families we have been blessed with. But the one thing that truly makes us "peas in a pod" is that we are passionate about helping guys to look and feel their best in the most doable, effective, and sustainable way possible.

Every guy's dream is to build muscle and lose fat, and this is what *Men's Health Total Fitness Guide 2008 Muscle Chow* is all about. Gregg knows what it takes to get that ripped look, and it makes sense to take advice from a guy whose livelihood depends on delivering the quintessential picture of health every day...365 days a year! Besides, Gregg is a National Academy of Sports Medicine–certified personal trainer and a *Men's Health* columnist whose expert advice over the years has helped lots of guys build the perfect body.

In this book, Gregg lays out the unique 2-month-cycle plan that he has designed and refined over his amazing career. He attributes his peak physical fitness to this effective and well-thought-out approach. Each orchestrated phase is designed with the sole purpose of achieving lasting results without having to swear off all of your favorite foods—forever! He eases you into it with a 1-week relaxed phase, revs it up a bit with a 5-week lean phase, and closes the deal with a more restrictive 2-week ripped phase that's guaranteed to get you the results you've always dreamed of. And you've got options. You say you don't care to be "ripped" and would be thrilled to just achieve "lean"? Skip the ripped part! But watch out—Gregg gives you a friendly kick in the butt and prods you to take the ripped phase for a little test run, just to see how it looks on you. He gives you the tools you need to achieve whatever level of fitness you desire.

There is brilliance in simplicity, truth, and enjoyment. *Men's Health Total Fitness Guide 2008 Muscle Chow* has them all. What attracted me to this book is its simplicity. What Gregg is asking you to do is not complicated, and the focus is on real food, smart workouts, and optimizing your results with select nutritional supplements. As a registered dietitian, it's important to me that my clients get a plan that's based on sound science and equally critical, produces results—*Men's Health Total Fitness Guide 2008 Muscle Chow* delivers on both! No wacky diet to be found here—no sir! Just the following well-founded principles:

Calorie balance is key.

Choose your calories wisely—and get filled up.

Pick the right proteins.

Muscles need lots of protein in order to grow, and *Men's Health Total Fitness Guide 2008 Muscle Chow* allows you to get your protein from a variety of delicious sources, with plenty of recipes for beef, chicken, turkey, egg, and seafood dishes. Gregg is an especially big fan of the most biologically available protein, whey. Whey not only delivers critical amino acids for quick muscle recovery and growth, but it also has been shown to build bones, improve your immune system, and even fight depression. Check out the protein shake recipes in Chapter 12.

Choose the right carbs. Gregg gets it right: You need a variety of both low- and high-glycemic-index foods, depending on what exercise and activities you're doing. This is not a "carb-phobic" plan! You'll find recipes for pasta and grains (Chapter 9); soups, veggies, and salads (Chapter 10); even biscuits and muffins (Chapter 11).

Fuel with the right fats. Not all fats are created equal. Want to recover faster after your workouts? Omega-3 fats smother the inflammation that results when you rip apart those muscles cells to prompt them to grow. Why be in pain any longer than necessary? Master the mouth-watering, muscle-building seafood recipes in Chapter 8.

Best of all, Gregg emphasizes the most important aspect of good, healthy food: *taste*! His delicious recipes have been taste-tested by his entire family.

Men's Health Total Fitness Guide 2008 Muscle Chow lays out a program to get you looking your best while increasing the odds that you, and maybe that someone special in your life, will enjoy your body for some time to come! Guess what? You are about to get *more* than you bargained for!

David Grotto, RD, LDN
Men's Health *nutrition advisor*
Author of 101 Foods That Could Save Your Life!
National Spokesperson, American Dietetic Association

INTRODUCTION

Achieving your best body ever is only possible when two elements merge as one—solid training and good nutrition. That's what *Men's Health Total Fitness Guide 2008 Muscle Chow* is all about. It's food for dudes, with more than 150 guy-friendly recipes to help you feed the beast. Much more than a cookbook, it explains how to tie together training and nutrition, helping you achieve your highest potential so you look your absolute best.

Most of us have no problem blitzing our muscles in the gym, but we struggle when it comes to maintaining a good diet. That's because a trip to the gym is a concentrated event with a beginning, middle, and end, helping you stay focused during your workouts. On the other hand, chowing food that's nutritionally sound is an all-day, everyday event that's constantly in your face. This makes it harder to consistently maintain a solid diet.

So let's put this into perspective. Guys ask me all the time how they can achieve a lean six-pack. Truth is, you can do crunches till the cows come home, but until you clean up your diet, you'll never have a good set of abs. This is where *Men's Health Total Fitness Guide 2008 Muscle Chow* comes in. It supports both your training and your nutritional habits by giving you a formula that actually works.

Over the past 10 years, I've become known as the *Men's Health* magazine cover dude who takes nutrition and supplementation very seriously. At every photo shoot, I sit down with everyone and talk about diet and supplements in a sort of round table. We discuss what the current trends are, how I prepared for the shoot, what I've been eating, why I've been eating it, and the supplements I'm using. Most people have the impression that I can eat whatever I want, train with moderate consistency, and still be able to shoot a cover at the drop of a hat. But if you ask anyone who knows me, especially the people at *Men's Health*, they'll tell you how dedicated and hardworking I am when it comes to health and fitness. I enjoy everything about it—the process of getting from one point to the next; the commitment, dedication, and consistency it takes to get there; and the feeling you get when you find the perfect balance that works. Above all, if there's one thing that people know about me, it's my sincerity and willingness to always help others discover their highest potential. That's how the "Muscle Chow" column evolved—from the reputation I earned over the years.

In the spring of 2006, *Men's Health* editor-in-chief David Zinczenko and I had an informal meeting over coffee to catch up. At the time, the "Muscle Chow" column had been running for two years with great success. If you've read the column, you know that Muscle Chow is "food with a function"—muscle food—designed to help you get the best possible results from all your hard work in the gym. David was thrilled with the feedback "Muscle Chow" had been receiving and encouraged me to consider writing a book based on the column.

Immediately the wheels in my head began turning. This was my opportunity to really help guys gain a better understanding of what to eat, when to eat it, and the easiest way to prepare it. Most of us are alike: We want food that's sensible, good tasting, quick to prepare, yet nutritionally sound to help us reach our goals. Beyond that, it seems like we're always searching for a plan to help us tie everything together—health, body, and mind. The Muscle Chow formula is one that I've spent years developing. It's a plan that allows you to harness these three elements so they work in your favor.

As I started putting my knowledge down on paper, I came to realize that this was valuable information that just can't be researched with your nose in a book and a pencil tucked behind your ear (or even via the vastness of the Internet). Through years of trial and error, I've experienced nutrition success firsthand—getting in the trenches, walking-the-talk to find what works and what doesn't, and applying it until I fine-tuned those principles. That's exactly what I've done for nearly three decades. So when you see me on a *Men's Health* cover, or on the cover of this book, you're looking at the culmination of knowledge I've gained—the same knowledge I offer to you now, in this book.

In the first chapter of the book, I offer a glimpse into my own personal journey, explaining the roots of Muscle Chow and the exact formula I now use to look my absolute best. I'll explain about 2-month healthy cycles, the three phases that make up each cycle, and how easy it is to integrate them into your daily regimen. The second chapter of the book features a shopping guide to help you organize your kitchen—fridge, pantry, cooking tools, and more—so grocery shopping and meal prep are a cinch.

Then we dive into the recipe chapter. This is the scope of my diet, from breakfast to dinner and all the snacks in between. It covers just about everything that I eat, explaining how to easily prepare meals for each of the diet phases.

In the final chapter of the book, you'll find a troubleshooting guide. This is a question-and-answer section to help assist you on your quest for your ultimate body.

Men's Health Total Fitness Guide 2008 Muscle Chow is a great resource that you'll want to keep handy, so go ahead, dog-ear the pages, make notes, get food stains on it—whatever. Use it and you'll finally achieve the results you've been looking for.

Before you turn to Chapter 1, I just want to get one last thing straight: This isn't brain surgery—it's learning how to eat more nutritionally dense foods as a way of life. That's it. There are no smoke and mirrors, no tricks up my sleeves—just basic clean eating for total wellness and, of course, for getting lean and shredded while adding dense muscle. The more you put in, the more you'll get out. Once you start, you'll begin seeing results in only a week. You'll feel leaner, with more energy, and immediately your workouts will improve. And by the time you finish your first cycle, you'll have a crystal clear understanding of why I use this formula—because it works! Now it's your turn. I'm in your corner, so let's get to it.

**EVERY RECIPE IN THIS BOOK IS DESIGNED TO HELP YOU
BUILD MUSCLE AND LOSE FAT.**

FEED YOUR MUSCLES

When it comes to seeing results from your workouts, there's nothing more important than your diet. You can pound the treadmill and lift weights from now to eternity and, at best, all that effort will contribute to only a fraction of the results you'll see. The rest comes from what you eat. Muscle fibers can't grow unless they're first broken down, so in essence, you lift weights to literally tear apart your muscles. To build them back up, you need nutrients. And the hows, whats, and whens of eating are crucial to making the sum of those two parts add up to 100 percent.

Believe me, maintaining a good clean diet—lean protein, nutritious fruits and vegetables, less sugary and salty junk food—is what separates the contenders from the pretenders. And that's what *Muscle Chow* is designed to do. Follow the plan, and this book will help you build the best body you can possibly achieve. It's that simple. When I eat the Muscle Chow way, I feel my best. I feel strong in and out of the gym. My mood is enhanced, which helps set the stage for killer workouts. I know I'm fueling my body well. Not only am I eating a diet that's designed to maximize my muscle-building potential, but I'm also keeping my body healthy. Study after study shows that diet plays a direct role in preventing heart disease, cancer, diabetes, Alzheimer's—you name it. Eating for muscle gain and for general good health don't have to be mutually exclusive. Muscle Chow gives you both.

If you were to ask any bodybuilder what the biggest key to his or her success might be, there's no doubt in my mind that the answer would be "diet." Working out is the easy part. Eating clean on a consistent basis is the tough part. That's because it takes discipline, and that's where *Muscle Chow* comes in.

WHAT MAKES MUSCLE CHOW DIFFERENT?

Let's look at the meaning of the word *diet*. It's defined as the average consumption of foods a person eats throughout life. Simply put, a diet should adapt to each individual and flow in an organic *balance* that's aligned with your environment and goals. If not, it doesn't feel right, and therefore will always seem like an uphill battle. And that's no way to eat. Too many diets exist in a vacuum; they assume conditions will always be perfect for you to eat one way forever, which is very unrealistic. They're all about the goal—the moment you arrive at the beach, the wedding, the reunion—but they never consider what happens after you reach the goal. The Muscle Chow plan is flexible; it's built around life's ups and downs to help create a balanced atmosphere for you and your individual goals.

Think of a swinging pendulum—the farther it swings in one direction, the farther it has to swing in the opposite direction. Training at your highest intensity without any kind of a break will ultimately lead to burnout and overtraining. The result can be anything from suffering an injury to putting your body in a catabolic state where your muscles stop growing. You begin going through the motions (or stop training altogether), and then you're faced with a setback. The same holds true for diet. If your eating is too restrictive for too long a period of time, you'll inevitably fall off the wagon and stop eating right—maybe even revert back to junk food. That's when fat starts accumulating, and again you're faced with a setback. Balance is what makes the Muscle Chow diet so successful, because you never allow that pendulum to swing so far in one direction that it comes back to knock you off your feet.

And Muscle Chow is more than simply turning you into a slab of lean beef. Sure, looking good is important. But so is feeling good. After all, what's the point of building a perfect body if you keel over from a heart attack at age 55? In addition to being lean, clean, muscle-building food, Muscle Chow is also healthy chow—full of quality lean proteins, the right fats and carbohydrates, plus the vitamins, minerals, and antioxidants you need to keep every system in your body primed.

THE KEYS TO A MUSCLE CHOW DIET

Do you sit down to every meal with a calculator in hand? No? Me neither. Any diet that requires more than basic counting skills is a diet that is way too complicated and will ultimately fail. Nutrition is a science, but it shouldn't have to be an agonizingly precise one. I've found that it's best to approach your diet with a relaxed attitude and not get bogged down by exact measurements of nutritional content. Make protein the starting point for each meal and snack—then surround it with a supporting cast of carbs and fat—it's that simple.

The following eight easy-to-remember strategies help me eat clean and meet those average percentages, without a lot of number crunching. They'll help you too. Think about it: If you increase your protein intake, something else has to decrease to compensate. (There's that balance principle again.) So if you trade a serving of carbs for a serving of protein, you've just doubled your protein intake while cutting your carbs by 50 percent. No calculator needed.

These are the strategies I use to help keep my diet in line.

1. EAT ENOUGH FOOD

Calories are your body's basic unit of energy. Everything your body does, from breathing to squeezing out that last rep, requires energy.

Here's a basic, yet effective way to determine your rough daily average caloric needs. I use this method myself and find that it's pretty darn accurate. Just multiply your body weight by 15. The total reflects the average caloric needs of an active male doing three or four cardio sessions weekly for 20 to 30 minutes each, and intense resistance training four or five days a week. So, to do the math: A 180-pound guy would need roughly 2,700 calories a day to maintain his body's energy balance.

Now, let's say you're not content to simply maintain your mass. If you want to build more muscle, you have to eat more. That can be hard to comprehend in a world where the evening news blares dire obesity warnings. But if you're training hard, like I know you are, you have to consume enough energy to support the muscle mass you're building. You have to add 3,500 calories to your weekly diet in order to gain a pound of muscle. Divide those calories over a week, and you need to add about 500 calories each day. (The reverse holds true as well: If you're trying to lose weight, you have to shave 3,500 calories out of your diet in order to drop a pound.)

That said, I've never been one to count every single calorie that I consume throughout the day. Sure, I have a ballpark idea, but realize that you're bound to consume more calories one day and fewer another. Remember that it's just as important to pay attention to the food choices you're making. If you expect to achieve strides in health and wellness, you've got to look at the integrity of the calories you're consuming. Empty carbs like white breads, cookies, fruit juices, and chips can't come close to the nutritional benefits of whole foods like vegetables, whole grains, and lean proteins. Which do you think will get you closer to your ultimate goal: chowing 600 calories of potato chips or 600 calories of broccoli? The way you choose to distribute those calories makes all the difference in the world to how your body will look and feel. By eating the Muscle Chow way, you can easily manage your weight to achieve the results you're looking for. Which brings us to the next strategy...

2. INCREASE YOUR PROTEIN INTAKE

If you're aiming to build muscle, you need more protein than the average couch potato. The people who know—such as the U.S. Olympic Committee and the American Dietetic Association—recommend 1.5 to 2.0 grams of protein per 2 pounds of body weight daily for athletes. That's more than double the U.S. government's recommended daily intake of 0.8 gram.

The reason? Exercise causes muscle damage. With every bicep curl you do, you're causing tiny tears in your muscle fibers. Protein helps repair those tears by providing the amino acids your body needs to form new cells—a process called protein synthesis. Amino acids repair the tears and fortify the fibers against future damage. The result: bigger muscles.

So to fuel the muscle-building process, you need plenty of protein. And not just immediately after your workout. One meal isn't enough to supply all the amino acids you need. Researchers from the University of Texas Medical Branch in Galveston have found that your body is primed for protein synthesis for up to two days after exercise. Protein—at breakfast, lunch, dinner, and in between—helps keep you in an anabolic state, during which your body creates more muscle protein than it breaks down. When your body can't keep up with the protein breakdown and repair cycle, you're in a catabolic state—not a good place to be if you're looking to create your best body.

As with calories, your need for protein increases as you build muscle mass, and because muscle tissues are metabolically active, things are constantly happening in

SHAKE THINGS UP

Can you get all the protein you need from food? Well, yes, I guess you could, but you'd probably be doing grocery store runs three times a day. This is where protein shakes come in handy—they're a fast, simple way to increase both your protein intake and your daily calories.

Protein mixes come in a seemingly endless array, but here's all you need to know: Choose a whey protein, casein protein, or a combination of both. In a Baylor University protein-supplement study, the combination of whey and casein protein promoted the greatest increases in fat-free mass after 10 weeks of heavy resistance training.

Whey, the liquid skimmed off during the cheese-making process, is the most readily absorbed protein source you can feed your body. It's quickly digested, which means it delivers amino acids to your muscles faster. It's particularly high in leucine, one of the branched-chain amino acids that helps you build bigger muscles. Whey also helps keep you feeling satisfied by releasing gut peptides that promote satiety. When University of Toronto scientists presented 22 men with an all-you-can-eat pizza buffet, the guys who had consumed a whey protein shake 2 hours earlier ate less of the pizza. You may feel like you could eat a horse after an intense gym session, but downing a whey shake will keep you clear of the stables.

Casein, another milk by-product, is also a high-quality protein, although it delivers amino acids more slowly. According to a study in the journal Human Nutrition and Metabolism, protein synthesis is three times greater with casein than with soy-based protein supplements. Soy is converted far more readily into urea, a waste product, and is eliminated during protein synthesis.

them. Twitch your leg, walk across the room, or turn a page of this book, and you've mobilized muscle tissues. Bench-press 225 pounds, and you've mobilized even more. Fat cells, on the other hand, just sit around your body waiting to be called up for duty in the event of a long stretch without food. As muscle grows and begins to displace fat cells, you need more protein to sustain it. For every pound of muscle added, you can burn between 50 and 75 extra calories a day—and that's a very good thing. In essence, as you build muscle, you're also creating a fat-burning machine!

Protein comes in more than one form. Here's some basic nutrition: There are 22 total amino acids, divided into essential (meaning they can only be obtained from diet), conditionally essential (meaning that your body can't synthesize them under certain conditions and that they too are best supplied by diet), and nonessential (meaning that your body can synthesize them without help from diet). Complete proteins are called complete because they contain all eight of the essential amino acids your body needs to repair cells. They're found in all animal products—red meat, poultry, dairy, and eggs.

Branched-chain amino acids (BCAAs) are a subcategory of essential amino acids, so named for their chemical structure. Fully a third of the amino acids found in your muscles are one of the three BCAAs: leucine, isoleucine, and valine. Intense training can deplete these, creating a demand for replenishment. Today, pure BCAAs are widely available in supplemental form (capsules, tablets, and powders). You can also find them in some postworkout recovery drinks, and most protein powders boast added BCAAs. The more readily available BCAAs are to your muscles during their repair phase, the more effectively protein is synthesized into those ripped muscle fibers.

Lean proteins like shellfish and turkey also provide B vitamins—thiamin, riboflavin, folate, and vitamins B6 and B12—that are especially important to the Muscle Chow diet. Your body needs B vitamins to convert proteins and sugars into energy, and to produce and repair cells. According to research from Oregon State University, athletes with low B vitamin levels are less able to repair and build muscle.

3. EAT HEALTHY FATS

When you're trying to gain muscle, fat can help. First of all, fat is the richest source of calories in the diet. One gram of fat contains 9 calories, versus 4 calories from a gram of either protein or carbs. Secondly, without enough fat, your body can't effectively produce testosterone, one of the key hormones for muscle growth. Go too low, and the way you look will be the least of your problems. Low testosterone levels can affect your sex drive, energy, vitality, mental focus, and overall sense of well-being.

But the primary benefit of fat is to your overall health. Unless you've been living under a rock for the past 20 years, you know that saturated fat—the kind you find in deep-fat fryers and animal meats (specifically fatty red meat)—has been linked to heart disease, strokes, and obesity. A particular subcategory of saturated fat—trans fat—has made headlines in recent years because it's even worse for your health. Trans fats are made by injecting vegetable oils with hydrogen to make them solid at room temperature, giving the junk foods they're found in life spans that would make a 500-year-old sequoia tree envious. On a calorie-for-calorie basis, trans fats increase heart disease risk more than any other nutrient (and I use the word *nutrient* only as a technical term—there's nothing nutritious about trans fats). Researchers have found that dietary levels of trans fats as low as 1 percent can raise the risk of heart disease by 23 percent. What's more, trans fats have also been shown to worsen arterial inflammation, one of the major risk factors for cardiovascular disease.

Monounsaturated and polyunsaturated fats have the opposite effect on your health: They boost your body's production of HDL, the "good" cholesterol, while lowering the bad stuff, LDL. They also help extinguish inflammation and keep your cell membranes and arteries supple. This is important for cellular communication, improved insulin sensitivity, and circulation. Avocados, most nuts, olives, olive oil, canola oil, and peanut oil are all good sources of monounsaturated fat. Cold-water fish, like salmon especially, and safflower, corn, and soybean oils are good sources of polyunsaturated fat.

Managing your dietary fat is an excellent example of how the well-balanced Muscle Chow approach works. If you choose lean sources of protein—poultry, fish, and lean beef—instead of cheeseburgers, sausages, and super-sized T-bones—you automatically cut some of the unhealthy fats out of your diet. Then, if you get rid of the junk carbs—ditch the baked goods and fried stuff and add in fruits, vegetables, nuts, and whole grains—you've removed even more. In the end, you'll create a shift from unhealthy fats to healthy fats, without even trying.

4. CHOOSE GOOD CARBS

If calories are the basic unit of energy, carbohydrates are the power lines that deliver fuel to your muscles. When you eat a carb—whether it's something starchy, like a potato; something sugary, like a piece of fruit; or something full of fiber, like whole grain bread—your body breaks it down into its elemental form: glucose, a type of sugar. Your pancreas produces a hormone called insulin to help carry glucose to cells throughout your body. The glucose is then converted to glycogen and stored in your muscles and liver. But if your muscles are full, excess glucose can be converted and stored as another energy source that's much harder to get rid of: fat. What's more, while the liver's storage capacity for glycogen is approximately 100 grams of carbs, your muscles hold approximately 400. But here's the kicker—there's no capacity limit for fat. In other words, if you need more storage space, your body just creates more fat cells. This is why managing your carb intake is smart nutrition. I'm not saying you need to go on a super low-carb diet; just be mindful of the macronutrient balance we spoke about earlier when you grab something to eat.

The type of carbs you eat affects the speed with which your body turns them into glucose. If you eat a starchy or sugary carb, your body turns it into glucose faster, supplying quick energy. Chow down a whole grain or something with a lot of fiber, and the glucose-conversion process slows down, supplying sustained energy.

CAN THE SOFT DRINK HABIT

Sodas have an average of 40 grams of sugar per 12-ounce can. That's pure glucose. And it comes with no redeeming vitamins. Diet soda is sweetened with artificial substances that are surrounded by controversy. All soda contains phosphates that leach essential nutrients like calcium from your body. If you're a soda drinker, you're probably saying you just can't give it up. But if you really want to, you can do it. Need a little help? Chew, or drink, on this: German scientists found that people who drank ice water increased their metabolic rate by 30 percent for up to an hour and a half. So grab an ice-cold one—a bottle of water, that is.

This is where the glycemic index (GI) comes in. Developed by Australian researchers, the glycemic index measures the rate of absorption that a certain carbohydrate has in the body, which in turn influences the release of insulin. The glycemic index ranks food based on a scale from 0 to 100; the higher a food rates on the index, the more it causes blood sugar—and, in turn, insulin—to rise. Doughy white bread is the easiest example to illustrate the point because it scores more than 70 on the glycemic index. White bread is made with just bleached flour and water. This means your system converts it into glucose very quickly. And if your glycogen stores are topped off, then the carb is converted to fat. Now, if you were to trade that plain white bread for a piece of grainy whole wheat bread—you know, the kind with nuts and seeds crusted all over the top—the conversion process would slow down, meaning that wheat bread rates lower on the glycemic index. Proteins and fats added to a carbohydrate-rich meal also help slow this conversion process, which is why the Muscle Chow diet adheres to a balance between these macronutrients.

Aside from being transformed into body fat, an overabundance of fast-converting carbs can also wear down your endocrine system. Each time your glucose levels rise, your pancreas has to pump out insulin to restore the balance. After years of overwork, you can become insulin resistant. Or even worse, your pancreas eventually goes on strike and that's when your doctor might hand you a diagnosis for type-2 diabetes—no matter how lean or cut you are.

So you should avoid high-GI carbs like the plague, right? Not necessarily. Here's the trouble with relying exclusively on GI. First of all, it's not intuitive. Until you have it memorized, you have to keep a list handy to know that a pear is low GI while a watermelon is high. Second, sometimes you need starchy or sugary high-GI carbs for energy.

For example, Gatorade ranks nearly at the top of the GI list, with a score of 91 out of 100. But that's the whole point of Gatorade: After a workout, it supplies glycogen-depleted muscles with much-needed energy and restores electrolytes you've sweated away. Third, GI fails to account for the other stuff you eat. Sure, a slice of bread is high GI. But top that slice with peanut butter or flaxseed oil—or any source of fat, protein, or fiber—and you've automatically cut the bread's GI.

Finally, I've met too many guys who miss out on the benefits of fruits, vegetables, and whole grains because they've been brainwashed against them. That watermelon you've been avoiding because of its high GI score (72) contains a nutrient called lycopene—nearly 30 percent of the amount that current research suggests helps to prevent prostate cancer. Plus, the melon acts as a diuretic, ridding you of subcutaneous water (H_2O between your skin and your muscles) and allowing you to look more cut the next day.

Again, I take a balanced approach. The real carbohydrate troublemakers are foods you know you shouldn't be eating much of anyway. Junk carbs—cookies, crackers, chips, pretzels, french fries—have no place in your diet, no matter if you're an Olympic athlete, a bodybuilder, or just a normal guy who's trying to replace his spare tire with a six-pack. These are the kinds of carbs that provide a quick jolt of energy by elevating your blood sugar. Every time you eat them, your pancreas sends out more insulin to help balance the glucose. Over time, the system goes berserk and your body can't handle the seesawing levels.

Avoiding junk carbs isn't rocket science, and it doesn't require much memorization either. If you can't easily trace a food back to its source in nature, don't eat it. Oats grow in fields; Oreos don't. Any healthy diet should make room for good carbs, and you should too.

5. EAT AT LEAST SIX SERVINGS OF FRUITS AND VEGETABLES EACH DAY

Unless they're baked into a sugary confection or breaded and fried in lard, fruits and vegetables are not the enemy. Do they contain carbs? Yes. Do you need to obsess about those carbs? No. If you expand your produce horizons beyond french fries and baked Idaho potatoes, you'll automatically help lower your meal's GI and cut out unnecessary fat. Plus, you'll gain a host of health and muscle-building benefits.

Your body is a complex system, and it can't run on protein and carbs alone. You

FORBIDDEN FRUIT

Juices sound like a healthy alternative when you're thirsty. Do yourself a favor, though, and check out the label next time you decide to have a tall glass. You might be surprised at the sugar it contains. The juice has been separated from the fruit's natural pulp, eliminating the fiber that slows your body's absorption of the food's sugar. So you're drinking a sugary liquid that your body quickly converts to glucose, sending your insulin levels through the roof. I'd much prefer that you drink bottled water and enjoy the full spectrum of a fruit's benefits by eating it whole.

need fiber to move food through your system, calcium to help fire the nerve cells that contract your muscles, potassium to help balance fluid levels and relieve muscle cramps, and a variety of antioxidants to help tamp down inflammation in your muscles after a tough workout. Fruits and vegetables contain vital nutrients not available in vitamin supplements. By eating these foods on a daily basis, you reap the benefits of all the naturally occurring nutrients they hold, helping lower your risk of cancer, heart disease, diabetes, and many other diseases.

Fruits and vegetables can also have a direct correlation to your ability to build muscle. Australian researchers found that men who cut their fruit and vegetable intake by just 1 serving for 2 weeks reported feeling they were exerting more effort when exercising. If you don't have enough B vitamins—like the folate found in leafy greens; the niacin found in bananas, peaches, and melon; or the full spectrum of Bs provided by avocados—you may lack energy and perform worse during high-intensity exercise.

Three servings of fruit and 3 servings of vegetables daily aren't that difficult to achieve. A single serving is equal to a medium piece of fruit, ½ cup of berries, 1 cup of raw leafy greens, or ½ cup of other veggies.

In my opinion, the two very best fruits and veggies are apples and broccoli. Apples satisfy your appetite any time of the day because they're high in both soluble and insoluble fiber. Insoluble fiber helps to move bulk through your system, while soluble fiber (pectin) helps to reduce cholesterol levels and slow down digestion. Try having an apple before a meal, like an appetizer (an apple-tizer!), to keep you from chowing too much in a single sitting, or have one as a snack between meals to help control your appetite.

Broccoli is the wonder veggie. Chewing and digesting broccoli consumes more calories than the veggie contains. A single stalk boasts about 3.5 grams of both fiber and protein, with as little as 6 grams of carbs and 350 milligrams of potassium. Since it's from the cruciferous family, broccoli is high in cancer-fighting indoles. It's also high in calcium, a mineral that helps to break down fats, and vitamin C to aid with recovery from a hard workout.

6. EAT LESS SALT

As a rule of thumb, I rarely add any salt to anything. According to the USDA, we don't need more than 500 milligrams daily. Most people get more than that amount for breakfast! Seriously. A slice of bacon can contain 1,000 milligrams. Read labels and notice the serving sizes—you might be floored by the amount of sodium some of your favorite foods contain. Too much sodium in your diet causes edema (water retention) and can make you look puffy. If that's not enough to make you limit sodium in your diet, consider this: It can also lead to high blood pressure and heart disease.

About 75 percent of the sodium we eat comes from processed food, not from the salt shaker. Frozen foods, canned foods, cured meats like bacon and sausage, fast foods, and sauces are some of the usual suspects. But even healthier foods like cottage cheese can contain high levels. You'll find that whenever possible, the Muscle Chow recipes call for low- or no-sodium ingredients, to help you avoid the excess.

When I do use salt, I use sea salt. Sea salt is obtained by the simple process of concentrating seawater under the sun. Up to 5 percent of sea salt is composed of naturally occurring potassium, calcium, and magnesium, the minerals that are responsible for the salt's mild flavor and good taste. Because sea salt is naturally occurring, your body can readily assimilate its minerals—they're just like the nutrients from food. Table salt, the salt most people use, is mined from inland salt deposits, heated to extremely high temperatures, and refined with chemicals. Potassium iodide or sodium iodide is added to create iodized salt. Dextrose (sugar), sodium bicarbonate, and sodium silico-aluminate are often added to keep the salt white and easy to pour.

7. TIME YOUR MEALS FOR MAXIMUM RESULTS

Muscles don't automatically inflate to Schwarzenegger-esque proportions just because you work out. Heck, that's only part of the equation. The other component is feeding the machine. You might spend an hour or two in the gym training hard to work your muscles and tear down muscle tissue, but then your body needs 48 to 72 hours to fully recover and heal. Part of that recovery—a big part—is paying attention to when you eat. When it comes to stimulating muscle growth, increasing mass, and ramping-up your metabolism, timing is everything.

Conventional nutritional wisdom has shifted from the three square meals a day that you probably grew up with to a series of smaller meals. So, instead of skyscraping peaks and rock-bottom lows, your body receives a steady stream of energy throughout the day. This lessens the burden on your endocrine system too. Since you're not ingesting huge floods of food at once, your pancreas doesn't have to pump out as much insulin to convert the food to glucose.

Multiple small meals also encourage your body to use calories rather than hoard them. When you go for long periods of time without food, you're sending a signal to your brain to start conserving energy. It's like turning down your body's thermostat. Your metabolism slows down. In this conservation mode, the system stores the nutrient yielding the highest calories per gram—fat. Fat yields 5 more calories per gram than either protein or carbs. So, by chowing every 2 to 3 hours, you keep your body in a state of liberation and your metabolism cooking.

The smaller-meals-more-often approach has other important Muscle Chow implications. First, there are those extra calories you need to consume in order to build muscle. Eating more often helps you get these calories effectively. No need to cram a side of beef down your pie-hole just to keep up with your caloric demand. Second, by avoiding energy deficits, your body stays anabolic longer. Make protein the centerpiece of those small meals and snacks, and you keep the pool of amino acids full and available for muscle repair. Your body needs those amino acids around the clock. Remember, the muscle repair process takes 48 to 72 hours.

Here's what I've found works the best: Make your main meals—breakfast, lunch, and dinner—smaller. Think two-thirds of a conventionally sized meal, then add snacks in between. I eat again approximately 2 hours after each meal and 3 hours after each snack. The lists on the next page give examples starting with breakfast at 7:00 a.m. If you're still hungry at 10:00 p.m., you can have a late snack that includes a slower-digesting casein protein to keep you anabolic longer into the night. (For ideas, check out some of the simple recipes using cottage cheese, in "Snacks" on page 23.)

WORKOUT DAY

7:00 a.m.: Breakfast

10:00 a.m.: Midmorning Snack

12:00 p.m.: Lunch

3:00 p.m.: Midafternoon Snack

5:00 p.m.: Preworkout Snack

6:30 p.m.: Postworkout Snack

8:00 p.m.: Dinner

10:00 p.m.: Evening Snack

NON-WORKOUT DAY

7:00 a.m.: Breakfast

10:00 a.m.: Midmorning Snack

12:00 p.m.: Lunch

3:00 p.m.: Midafternoon Snack

5:00 p.m.: Late-afternoon Snack

7:00 p.m.: Dinner

10:00 p.m.: Evening Snack

Schedule your meals and snacks around your workouts. Eating about 30 minutes to an hour before a workout gives you the energy you need to lift. You wouldn't expect your car to run if the gas tank was empty, would you? This is your chance to not only set the stage for optimum muscle gains but also enhance your fat-burning potential.

If you work out in the morning, make time for a quick breakfast before you hit the gym. A protein shake mixed with water (my choice) or fat-free milk will break your fast and ensure your body stays anabolic by feeding your hungry muscles with the amino acids they need to grow on. The best choice here would be a fast-digesting protein (like whey) with little to no added fat, carbs, or sugar. The lack of carbs will allow your body to target fat much quicker than if you had fully plumped glycogen stores. If you still need energy to help motivate and drive you into the gym, have some caffeine. A cup of coffee will help raise your metabolism, increase your energy levels, and support your fat-burning potential as well.

People who, like me, find that their hunger pangs can get in the way of a solid workout need to chow something beforehand. For those individuals, having some fruit can be the answer. Eat an apple, a pear, a peach, a couple slices of cantaloupe, or a handful of strawberries, raspberries, or blueberries. The carbs in the fruit will help give you extra energy for your workout.

If you train later in the day (like I do), chances are you'll have already eaten several times by then, so your glycogen stores will be nice and full. Since you probably don't need to fuel your system anymore at this point, stick with a protein shake mixed with water or fat-free milk. For more preworkout snack ideas, see "Pre-Pump Foods" on page 201. If you're still lacking motivation to hit the gym, swing by a coffee joint to down a shot of espresso or chug an energy drink.

Eating after a workout is a touch more complicated because it involves manipulating one of your body's most powerful hormones—insulin. Immediately after your last rep, muscles are primed for a glycogen infusion. Their glycogen stores are empty, and it's a green light to chow. Eat carbohydrates, especially fast-converting carbs like bread or a high-carb energy drink, and your muscles will suck them up like a sponge. That's because those high-GI carbs trigger the release of insulin to help carry glucose directly to muscle cells, where it's socked away as glycogen. This is a window of opportunity I never miss, and it lasts for about an hour, then diminishes every minute thereafter.

Replenishing your body with high-GI carbs postworkout can also help enhance the effects of certain supplements—notably creatine, which you'll learn more about on page 16. Carbs are the engine that drives creatine directly into the muscle cells. They also aid in protein synthesis, especially after exercise when amino acids are in high demand and your muscles are looking to begin the process of rebuilding. Based on my own experience and all the well-documented research, I can't emphasize enough the importance of providing your muscles with these lost nutrients as soon as possible after you work out. For postworkout meal ideas, see "Recovery Foods" on page 224.

8. KEEP A LOG

I use a food journal every day to keep track of exactly what and when I need to feed the beast. This accomplishes three things:

1. You can quickly determine when you should (or can) eat your next meal or snack. Remember, eat snacks 2 hours after each meal and meals 3 hours after each snack.

2. You become accountable for everything you eat. If you have to write down every bite in your food journal, you'll think twice before you chow on something that isn't good for you.

3. You also can quickly calculate ballpark figures of total protein and carbs for the day, using the nutrition info that accompanies each Muscle Chow recipe or the

SAMPLE DAILY FOOD LOG

TIME	FOOD(S)	PROTEIN	CARBS	CALORIES (OPTIONAL)
7:00 a.m.	Toast with whole fruit preserves	11 g	45 g	230
	90% Shake	50 g	10 g	216
10:00 a.m.		–	20 g	70 g
Totals:				

Nutrition Facts panel on labels of packaged foods. Again, you don't need to be exact in your calculations, so long as you have a basic idea.

I've provided a sample log page above and on page 278. Just run off some photocopies and you're all set!

CYCLING THROUGH PHASES

At the beginning of this chapter, I briefly spoke about the Muscle Chow plan and how this book will help you build the best body you can possibly achieve. Sure, the recipes alone will get you leaner and help you build muscle, but here's where it all comes together. Using the eight strategies we just outlined as a general guideline, I maintain my dietary strategies within 2-month cycles. These cycles are the secret to my success. They help make setting and reaching goals very accessible, plus they help maintain consistency—a key component for success. Each cycle starts off relaxed, and as the cycle progresses, dietary restrictions are tightened. (Think of it like a good book or movie with a beginning, middle, and end.) Each 2-month cycle is divided into three phases: a Relaxed Phase, a Lean Phase, and a Ripped Phase.

The Relaxed Phase lasts 1 week and is the least restrictive. Basically you're off your diet and taking a break. The Lean Phase (I also call this my maintenance diet) adds some restrictions. It lasts 5 weeks and is a "clean" diet with lots of lean protein, complex carbs, and healthy fats. The Ripped Phase kicks it up another notch, with fewer calories and starchy carbs. It lasts the final 2 weeks before falling back into a Relaxed Phase. The Ripped Phase is the most restrictive portion of a 2-month cycle and can really set you apart as you zero in on your goals. Once you string a couple of these 2-month cycles together, you'll see how maintaining a well-balanced diet becomes easy. There are no hard falls because you never allow the pendulum to swing too far in one direction.

RELAXED PHASE: 1 WEEK

While any of the recipes in this book are perfectly acceptable for the Relaxed Phase of a diet cycle, this is your opportunity to indulge your craving for foods that are outside the parameters of Muscle Chow. Treat yourself to pizza, a fast-food meal, or just more carbs than usual—like cereal, granola and fruit bars, breads, and pasta. On average, calories are at their highest in a Relaxed Phase.

RELAXED SPECS

Drink one protein shake daily. The morning hours from breakfast to lunch, when your muscles are primed for replenishment, are a great time for a whey shake. You can mix this shake with water, fat-free milk, or soy milk—it's up to you.

Begin a creatine-loading cycle (optional). If you're not ready to use supplemental creatine, that's okay, but the benefits of creatine are well known. I don't believe any other sports supplement has as much proof to support its use. In countless studies, creatine has been shown to increase gains in muscle mass and strength by providing more energy to your muscles during exercise. It also helps hydrate muscle cells, giving you more muscle volume. In fact, some creatine products can increase muscle volume and total body weight by as much as 7 to 10 pounds in as little as a week. I know that sounds crazy, but it's true.

Today, there are so many different creatine products on the market that it can make your head spin. New forms of creatine and creatine products seem to emerge on a monthly basis. And one thing's for certain: They'll continue to do so as long as this product sits atop the muscle-building mountain. Most of these new creatine products—creatine ethyl ester (CEE), creatine alpha-ketoglutarate (AKG), Kre-Alkalyn, creatine gluconate, and dicreatine malate—claim better absorption than basic creatine monohydrate, while causing less water retention. Numerous studies show that consuming creatine with a simple carbohydrate (instead of water) enhances the absorption by 20 percent to 40 percent. That's why many creatine products come premixed with dextrose (a form of sugar) or some other kind of carbohydrate. You can also mix plain micronized creatine monohydrate into sweetened tea, sport drinks, or applesauce to achieve the same effect.

Usually a creatine cycle starts with what's called a loading phase. This is designed to saturate your muscles with creatine. How much is a loading dose? That varies on the creatine you buy, but the average is 20 to 30 grams per day.

Creatine supplements are much more efficient than trying to get creatine from food. Most animal proteins contain approximately 2 grams of creatine per pound. When you think about it, a pound is a lot of fish, beef, or fowl to be choking down just to get a couple grams of creatine. It's easier to pop creatine into a shake. Plus, supplements may be easier to time. I've gotten my best results by consuming creatine midmorning on nontraining days and immediately postworkout on training days. You want to supply creatine to your muscles postworkout, when they are starving for glycogen replenishment.

Take a multivitamin/mineral. This one's simple. Taking a multivitamin/mineral is like having an insurance policy for your body. It gives you blanket coverage just in case your diet isn't 100 percent perfectly calibrated to deliver all of the vitamins, minerals, and antioxidants you need. In fact, I don't know too many people who get all their daily nutrients from foods alone. Unless you're cultivating your own fruits and veggies, and making everything from scratch using whole grains and unprocessed ingredients, taking a multivitamin/mineral supplement is a good idea.

Now what does a good multi do for us guys who train hard? After all, this is Muscle Chow. First, vitamins and minerals are involved in every metabolic contraction, exertion, and dilation that takes place in response to each movement you make. Let's go another step and talk about those last few burning reps associated with muscle fatigue.

That burning sensation is a buildup of lactic acid in the muscle, the by-product of your muscles converting glycogen to energy—a process called glycolysis. This causes an increase in circulation to help flush lactic acid from blitzed muscles and aid in recovery between sets. That, along with the cardio aspect of training, produces an increase of oxygen in the blood. In turn, this also increases the opportunity for oxidative stress and the formation of free radicals, unbalanced molecules that can mess with the DNA in your cells. Whew, you still with me? In a nutshell, antioxidants help get rid of those free radicals before they can cause harm. So you can see the importance of a multivitamin containing essential antioxidant vitamins like C, E, beta carotene, and selenium.

I recommend that you take a multi that's specifically formulated for men. Guys don't need the excess iron and vitamin A that can be found in generic multis.

Training suggestion: Train with moderate to high intensity 3 to 4 days this week. Cardio is an option in the Relaxed Phase.

LEAN PHASE: 5 WEEKS

Here's where you get in the trenches and really pay attention to diet and training—a combination that increases lean body mass and strength while reducing unnecessary fat. When you hear the term *eating clean,* this is it. Just about every recipe in this book (and foods with comparable nutritional values) are appropriate for the Lean Phase. However, the comfort foods that you've been chowing in the Relaxed Phase—like pizza, for instance—will have to wait for another 7 weeks.

LEAN SPECS

Concentrate on protein intake. As your training intensifies, so does your body's need for protein. It's important to get a serving of lean protein (in the form of food or a shake) at every main meal and snack.

Drink two protein shakes daily. Because the Lean Phase emphasizes macronutrient balance, you're chowing protein all day long. That means you can pick any time of the day to down a shake in place of eating protein. You may choose to have your shakes when you want quick assimilation, like pre- or postworkout, but it's up to you.

Eat one higher-carb meal per week. This helps satisfy cravings, helps keep your metabolism ramped up, and makes your muscles look nice and full. An extra serving of pasta, brown rice, or sweet potatoes are all great choices.

Add 5 grams of L-glutamine supplement twice daily. L-glutamine is one of the most important amino acids for guys who are physically active and want to keep themselves in peak condition. That's because it's one of the most abundant amino acids found in every muscle in the body. Upon extreme physical activity, your body draws large amounts of L-glutamine from the most abundant source you have—muscles. Therefore, a lack of this important amino acid can lead to muscle breakdown (aka catabolism).

Glutamine is best used throughout the day in small doses, rather than in one big dose. Many of the Muscle Chow foods you'll consume daily, like salmon, spinach, and cottage cheese, help replenish glutamine. For example, a 6-ounce can of tuna and a cup of cottage cheese contain around 3 grams of L-glutamine each; a handful of almonds contains about 1 gram; and whole grain toast contains about ½ gram (500 milligrams) per slice. By consuming a balanced diet of fresh veggies, lean meats, fish, and dairy, you'll ensure you're getting a good dose of natural L-glutamine from those foods to help with muscle recovery. Muscle Chow recipes that are chock-full of L-glutamine include Loaded Spinach Salad on page 174, the salmon dishes in Chapter 8, Loaded Soup on page 153, and the beef recipes in Chapter 4. If you're looking for an added boost, protein shakes and L-glutamine powders are widely available. Supplementing with L-glutamine can help maintain muscle integrity, support immune function, and aid in muscle recovery—all the things needed to build a better body. To ensure my body has the glutamine it needs, I take 5 grams of glutamine 30 minutes pre- and postworkout. If it's been a hardcore training day, I'll have another 5-gram dose before bed.

Take 1,000 milligrams of an essential fatty acid (EFA) supplement twice daily. There are two subcategories of dietary fat that are essential: omega-3 and omega-6 fatty acids. *Essential* means that they cannot be produced by the body and therefore need to be supplied by the diet. Studies show that the average American consumes more omega-6s than omega-3s, from foods like grains, breads, poultry, and eggs. Maybe that's because omega-3–rich foods take a little more effort to chow. I'm talking about fish like salmon, tuna, and sardines; flaxseeds and flaxseed oil; nuts; soybeans (edamame) and other legumes; and olive oil. It's important to get a balance of these two essential fatty acids in your diet for proper health, so increasing your intake of omega-3s becomes a priority. The Muscle Chow recipes can help, but it's still a good idea to take a good EFA supplement to ensure you reap all the health benefits these amazing fats have to offer.

The types of omega-3 fatty acids you need are called eicosapentaenoic acid (EPA) and docosahexaenoic acid (DHA). Don't worry, you don't have to spell them—just eat them. These are the two principal fatty acids found in fish, and they're the most readily available omega-3s used by the body. Recent research has linked them to everything from reduced risk of heart disease to increased intelligence. When scientists compared the IQ levels of 300 people tested in 1947 with a 2001 follow-up, they found that those who had consumed fish oil supplements outperformed earlier tests by 13 percent. Not only do these fatty acids help your brain's processing speed, they have a host of Muscle Chow benefits. Researchers from the University of Western Ontario have found that omega-3s help you shed body fat while gaining muscle. They help you handle insulin more efficiently, stoke your metabolism on a cellular level, reduce inflammation, discourage your body from storing fats, and help keep your hormones optimized. They also lube your joints, which is helpful when you're on that third set of squats and your knees are feeling the pressure. Since many health-conscious guys try to achieve the perfect six-pack by maintaining low-fat diets, supplementing with EFAs is especially important.

You can easily find EFA supplements at any health food store in flavored liquids for palatability or in gel capsules. Because omega-3 supplements are made from fish oil, they can sometimes make you belch a fishy aftertaste. To avoid it, be sure to consume them with food.

Reduce your creatine supplementation to a maintenance level. If you decided to start taking creatine in the Relaxed Phase, it's time to decrease your dosage to between 5 and 15 grams daily. This maintenance dose should last throughout the entire 2-month cycle. If you decide to continue taking creatine through the next 2-month cycle, don't do the loading phase again—rather, continue with the maintenance dose. At the end of a second consecutive 2-month cycle, take a break from creatine supplementation for a full 2-month cycle before starting again (beginning with a loading phase).

Continue taking your multivitamin/mineral. Once you're in the Lean Phase, you may find that you want to stick with it all the time. Theoretically, you could—but let's not get carried away. "All the time" is a very long time. Eating just one way forever is a strategy that can set you up for failure. I always suggest you begin with a complete 2-month cycle in the proper order—start with the Relaxed Phase and have some of those foods you might be craving, then move into the Lean Phase where you maintain a clean diet, and finally go into the Ripped Phase to get super lean.

After one full cycle, you might decide to forgo the Relaxed Phase for your next 2-month cycle and start directly back into a Lean Phase diet. That's okay if you choose to do so, but consider enjoying a Relaxed Phase the next time it comes around (8 weeks later). The idea of eating in phases is to maintain balance and to keep that pendulum from swinging too far in one direction. It's just like changing up your workout—it keeps your body guessing and adapting, while also keeping things fresh and interesting.

Training suggestion: Train with high intensity 4 to 6 days a week. Do cardio 3 to 4 days a week, at moderate to high intensity.

RIPPED PHASE: 2 WEEKS

I consider these final two weeks of a 2-month cycle to be a pre-photo-shoot diet, although it doesn't require you strap on a slingshot bikini and stand in front of a camera. Here's where you tighten the diet and punch up the intensity of your training a notch. On average, calories are at their lowest because the food choices are so clean. Use this phase to get ready for any situation where you want to look your absolute best: a beach vacation, cruise, wedding, reunion, or just to achieve a personal goal and feel your best. To accomplish this, you'll need to stick with the recipes in this book that have a Ripped Phase icon (or foods with comparable nutritional values) during these final two weeks. The good news is that you can also eat any of the Ripped Phase recipes at any point during an entire 2-month cycle.

Some people might find the Ripped Phase too restrictive. If so, you might decide not to go into a Ripped Phase on your first cycle, but don't give up on it. I believe this final phase can be your crowning moment that proves you can achieve your ultimate physique. If you choose not to go into the Ripped Phase, continue the Lean Phase for another two weeks until you've completed a 2-month cycle. At that point it will be time to fall back into a Relaxed Phase (and grab a cheat meal or two) as the next 2-month cycle begins.

RIPPED SPECS

Drink three protein shakes daily. The extra protein helps replace some of the carbs you're cutting. Midafternoon and evening snacks are good times to chug a shake because they will help you feel satiated as your overall calories are reduced. Post-workout is also an important time—it's your window of opportunity to feed hungry muscles.

Prepare only recipes that have a Ripped Phase icon (or foods with comparable nutritional values). Note that a few recipes require tweaks to make them suitable for a Ripped Phase. Look for the "Ripped Tip."

Eat only lean white-meat proteins such as chicken, fish, turkey, and eggs. This

RIPPED RECIPES

The following recipes carry a Ripped Phase icon designating them as appropriate meal choices during a Ripped Phase of a 2-month Muscle Chow diet cycle.

helps minimize your saturated fat intake to help get you ripped, while still providing high-quality lean protein. None of this book's beef recipes, in Chapter 4, carry a Ripped Phase icon.

Eat one–and only one–pasta meal during this 2-week period. Do this in the second week of a Ripped Phase to help fill muscles with glycogen. Glycogen is stored via water, so it helps muscles become nice and full. This action also pushes subcutaneous veins to the surface of your skin, so you look more vascular—especially in the final stages of a 2-month cycle. For this meal, you may choose from any of the Pastas & Grains recipes (Chapter 9), though only one of those recipes, Protein-Rich Quinoa Salad, features a Ripped Phase icon.

Avoid baked goods. None of the Biscuits & Muffins recipes (Chapter 11) are appropriate for a Ripped Phase.

Desert dessert. Desserts (Chapter 14) are devoid of Ripped Phase icons. There are plenty of Ripped Phase snacks to indulge in, however.

Drink eight (16-ounce) bottles of water a day. When you work out more, you sweat more, so the extra H_2O keeps you hydrated.

Continue to:

- Take a multivitamin/mineral daily
- Take 5 grams of L-glutamine supplement twice daily
- Take 1,000 milligrams of essential fatty acids (EFAs) twice daily
- Supplement with creatine daily

Training suggestion. Train with high intensity 4 to 6 days a week, while trying to increase the amount of weight you're lifting (pay attention to proper form). Do high-intensity cardio 3 days a week.

Unless you're a seasoned veteran in health and fitness and you already maintain a clean diet, jumping headlong into the Ripped Phase without moving through the first two phases is something I don't recommend. The Muscle Chow formula is one that I've been doing for a long time, and I have found that the best results are achieved through patience and consistency. Switching from a carefree diet to a highly restrictive diet overnight will be more difficult than you think. Start slow and work your way up.

As for staying in the Ripped Phase for longer than two weeks, again keep in mind that this phase is very restrictive, so you can become extremely burned out if you do it for too long (remember the swinging pendulum). It's great to look your best today and into next week, but it's just as important to look your best four months from now and into next year. No doubt—a Ripped Phase type diet will give you dramatic results. Just don't climb to the top of the hill without realizing how far down the valley might be on the other side.

THE CYCLE IS OVER—NOW WHAT?

At the end of a 2-month cycle, it's time to begin the next cycle, starting again with the Relaxed Phase. Enjoy yourself; after 7 weeks of consistency, you've earned 7 days to kick back a little. It's important not to fall off the wagon completely by super-sizing every day at the local fast-food joint and sucking down 40-ounce milkshakes. Opt for a few cheat meals and snacks here and there, while still trying to maintain balance in your diet. In other words, don't completely abandon fruits, veggies, whole grains, and protein. That way, it's not such a chore to get back on track when it's time to start the Lean Phase again (the next level of dietary restrictions).

You may decide you're not ready and want to stick with the Relaxed Phase for another week. That's okay; just be sure not to let an extra week turn into three weeks or a month. For this reason, I suggest marking your Lean Phase start date on a calendar with a highlighter (see "Getting Started" on page 26). If you make the commitment and write it down, you'll be accountable.

You can choose to set a new goal for each 2-month cycle, but it's not necessary. It's true that the most effective strategy for progress and growth is setting strong goals, but that doesn't mean you've got to change it every two months. A goal could take as long as a year to attain (six back-to-back cycles), while another might take four months (two back-to-back cycles). The key is having a strong vision—so strong that it motivates you to pursue your goal all the way to the end, no matter how long it takes.

HOLD ON A SEC...

Before you launch into a total diet overhaul, take a minute. Success in anything—whether it's a job, a hobby, a workout, or an eating plan—boils down to three words that I call the Big 3: **commitment**, **dedication**, and **consistency**.

The first—**commitment**—is your decision to make a change. The choice to better yourself, and your commitment to that choice, are big responsibilities. So often people float through their days, their weeks, their lives, afraid to make a commitment. The possibility of failure looms over our heads, and in turn, our willpower weakens. Sure, I've had my share of hard knocks—we all have. But I learned from those mistakes and picked myself up. Through it all, there is one thing that I never did—I never gave up. It's as simple as that.

Once you make the decision to change, emphasis shifts to the second component of the Big 3: **dedication**. Here you set the wheels in motion and dedicate yourself to a goal. This means getting rid of old habits and implementing new, more inspiring ones that will immediately start making a difference in your life. It takes perseverance to stick to new changes, especially when things get tough. Ultimately it's your choice: Push forward to new ground or fall back on old, comfortable habits. The consequences of that choice will either drive you closer to or pull you farther away from your goals.

When it comes to realizing your goals, the last of the Big 3 is probably the most important: **consistency**. When I think back over the years, this has to be the one that helped me the most. You know when your training is subpar, because you lack energy and motivation. You feel it the moment you enter the gym, during your workout, and walking out of the gym. You might rationalize, "Oh well, tomorrow's another day, the gym was crowded, I couldn't get on all the machines I wanted, my mind just wasn't into it, work was tough...." Yeah, and don't forget high gas prices, pollution, and global warming! The truth is that there's just no room for excuses. You can find a million reasons why you should skip the gym or put off eating a Muscle Chow diet until Monday, or next week, or even next month. But if you want to be your best, you've got to commit yourself to that cause and stick with it. Most people can't or won't maintain this level of consistency. It's not easy, and if it was, everyone would be doing it, right? That's why it feels so great when you put forth the effort and begin seeing results.

GETTING STARTED

You'll find that once you make a commitment and dedicate yourself fully, it will change your world. You've got to start by realizing you have the power to wipe the slate clean and become the architect of your future. There are no boundaries to your potential, no limitations to what you can achieve. Here's a three-step road map to achieving your best body.

Step 1: Have a vision. Create a clear picture of what you want out of your 2-month cycle. This simple task will set a point of reference to show you exactly where you're headed. This is one of the biggest issues for most of us. We lose sight of our vision too easily and end up falling off the wagon, only to beat ourselves up over it later.

The key is to find something that inspires you. It can be your high school football picture, when your body was at its best, a magazine photo of a physique you admire, or even a picture of the cruise ship you'll be vacationing on. Whatever it is, whoever it is, get a picture and tape it where you're going to see it every single morning (like on the inside of the kitchen cabinet where you keep the coffee mugs). When you see it, see yourself and restate your goal.

Step 2: Get a map. If you don't know where you're going, how the heck are you going to get there? Some people don't worry about that part. They jump in with both feet and deal with the details later. That's a formula for disaster. Each 2-month cycle is the framework—now you need a map to fill in the plan that will help you reach your goal. In my case, a calendar is my map. It's easy to print off a couple months from the computer (that's what I do), or just buy a calendar. Using a highlighter, mark a box around the first week in blue (Relaxed Phase), the next five weeks in yellow (Lean Phase), and the final two weeks in orange (Ripped Phase), until you've got it broken down into three blocks of time.

Step 3: Get started. You've got your vision, your goal, and your map—now it's time to get started. Two-month cycles are a formula that works—they've worked for me over the years, and they will work for you. These cycles ease you into the idea of eating a clean diet on a consistent basis. If you go balls-to-the-wall, you're going to set yourself up for a binge-eating blowout. The Relaxed Phase gets you ready, the Lean Phase helps you build consistency to achieve the best possible results in a relatively short period of time, and the Ripped Phase can help you reach that ultimate goal. Sure, the changes to your diet and a new training regimen might be tough at first, but you're embarking on an inspiring journey in the right direction.

2

READY, SET, COOK

Maintaining a diet that allows you to get lean while feeding your muscles the proper nutrition for growth can be tricky. That's where the following recipes will help you. I'm confident that you'll find the right mix of Muscle Chow recipes to fit your lifestyle; I've worked diligently to craft them. Some took me as many as a dozen or more tries before I got them perfect. Others have been staples in my diet for years, and I could probably make them with my eyes closed. If there's one thing I'm certain about, it's that Muscle Chow is sensible food that's easy to make. It's not gourmet or complex, yet some of the recipes can still make you look like a culinary connoisseur. As you go through them, you'll find a lot of valuable bits of information: cooking shortcuts, pre- and postworkout meals, quick snack suggestions, and tips on preparing food without a lot of mess. In fact, none of the recipes require a food processor (since it can be a pain to clean up), and I always try to use as few pots and pans as possible. This is simple cooking, with easy-to-understand steps and minimal prep times, so putting together a well-balanced meal plan can fit into anyone's busy schedule.

Are these recipes all the food you have to eat? Absolutely not. I always encourage people to incorporate their own recipes and favorite healthy foods using the key Muscle Chow principles on page 3 as a starting point. Unhealthy trans fats, empty carbohydrates, excess sugar, and hidden sodium are in more foods than you might imagine, which means you've got to sidestep nutritional land mines every time you hit the grocery store. Do your homework—take the time to read labels, check the Nutrition Facts chart, and scan the list of ingredients. Before you know it, you'll have your own array of healthy food choices along with your favorite Muscle Chow recipes to help you achieve great results.

THINGS YOU'LL NEED IN THE MUSCLE CHOW KITCHEN

Use these checklists to stock your fridge and kitchen cabinets. Keep the following items on hand, and you can make just about every recipe in this book.

IN THE FRIDGE

- ☐ **Large omega-3-fortified eggs:** These eggs, which you can find in just about every supermarket, come from free-range chickens raised without any drugs, hormones, antibiotics, or animal by-products. Studies show that free-range chickens, which eat a diet rich in pasture greens and insects, produce eggs with higher omega-3s than eggs from ordinary grain-fed chickens. That's because they're pecking natural grains and chowing insects. In addition, fortified eggs also contain higher amounts of antioxidants like vitamins A and E, and carotenoids—plus folic acid for protein metabolism and energy production. So be sure to check them out the next time you're in the egg section of your grocery store. They might be a little more expensive, but they're worth it, because omega-3 fatty acids help with muscle inflammation, enhance the body's ability to store glycogen, and improve the effectiveness of carnitine to help you burn fat more efficiently. Omega-3s also help increase your metabolism and improve your fat-burning potential. Store the eggs on a shelf in the refrigerator and not in the door, which is the warmest spot in the fridge. Use them within a month.
- ☐ **Fat-free plain yogurt**
- ☐ **No-salt cottage cheese**
- ☐ **Fat-free milk**
- ☐ **Low-sodium 100 percent whole grain bread:** Two of my all-time favorite bakery companies, and the ones I recommend when a recipe calls for bread, are Food For Life and Alvarado St. Bakery. Their products are made from organic

sprouted grains and other organic ingredients (including nuts and seeds). All their baked goods are made from whole grains and are lower glycemically than most others you'll find at the grocery store. Plus they're free of trans fats. My favorite bread from Food For Life is the Ezekiel 4:9 Organic Sprouted 100% Whole Grain Flourless Bread. I buy the low-sodium version because it tastes just as good as the regular, yet it contains almost no sodium. This company's breads are considered a complete protein, meaning they contain all eight of the essential amino acids that the body can't produce on its own. This is due to the combination of protein-rich grains and legumes (beans). Food For Life also carries a full line of whole grain hamburger and hot dog buns, as well as tortillas and pocket breads. The Alvarado St. varieties I most recommend are the No Salt! Sprouted Multi-Grain Bread (with only 10 milligrams of sodium per slice), the tasty Sprouted Soy Crunch Bread, and the Essential Flax Seed Bread. The company also offers a variety of other baked products, including rolls, buns, and bagels.

- ☐ **Fresh vegetables**
- ☐ **Fresh and frozen fruit**
- ☐ **100% whole fruit preserves**
- ☐ **Ground flaxseeds:** Once whole flaxseeds are ground, they need to be kept in the fridge in an airtight container. If not, they will spoil quickly.
- ☐ **Fat-free pump-spray butter:** Look for it in the supermarket dairy case. It's great on muffins, toast, pancakes, and sweet potatoes.
- ☐ **Soy lecithin granules:** Soy lecithin is probably best known as a nutrient that helps prevent arteriosclerosis and cardiovascular disease. Lecithin helps with cholesterol by shuttling excess fats from the body. It's also good for brain function, energy, and vascularity. Lecithin is an emulsifier, meaning that even though it's a fat, it doesn't repel water the way oil does. Instead, it's soluble in water, so you can add lecithin granules to protein shakes (see Chapter 12) and other recipes, such as Vein-Poppin' "Tapioca" Pudding on page 213, to help add more texture and thickness. You can find soy lecithin granules at any health food store.
- ☐ **Grated Parmesan cheese**
- ☐ **Frozen shelled edamame:** These soybeans are a good source of complete protein and L-glutamine, a nutrient that helps with muscle recovery and repair.
- ☐ **Fat-free ricotta cheese**
- ☐ **Fat-free sour cream**

- ☐ **Wheat germ:** With its mild nutty flavor, wheat germ can be sprinkled onto breakfast cereals and added into baked goods (such as the ones in Chapter 11) to help boost the nutritional profiles of those foods. It's a good source of vitamin E and folate—two antioxidants that help with energy production, cellular health, and immune function. It also contains other B vitamins and minerals such as selenium, magnesium, and zinc for a host of benefits including antioxidant health, glucose metabolism, and hormone production. Because of its high vitamin E content, wheat germ can spoil, so I always keep it in a jar in the fridge so it stays fresh. (Be sure to check the expiration date before using it.)
- ☐ **All-natural or sugar-free maple syrup**
- ☐ **Tofu:** Derived from soybeans, tofu is a rich source of complete proteins— meaning it contains all of the eight essential amino acids. This makes it a good option in your quest to find foods that support the muscle-building process. It is low in calories and saturated fats, has no cholesterol, and is easily digestible. Because soy contains phytoestrogens (plant estrogens), you might wonder if it can cause increased estrogen levels—and, therefore, cause lower testosterone levels and related side effects such as loss of muscle mass, increased body fat, reduced sex drive, gynecomastia (male breast enlargement), and enlarged prostate. Generally, the amount of estrogen you get from soy products is not large enough to be significant, according to Eric Sternlicht, PhD, a member of the American College of Sports Medicine. "It might become a factor if someone were eating soy as their exclusive source of protein—like somebody who's getting 100 to 150 grams of protein daily from soy products," says Sternlicht. So while chicken, fish, beef, and eggs are the main Muscle Chow proteins, tofu is a viable plant-based protein that can be included in your diet once or twice a month.
- ☐ **Apple butter**

IN THE PANTRY

- ☐ **Cooking sprays:** Because I use them just about every day, I like to keep a few different cooking sprays in the cupboard at all times. They're a super handy tool for low-fat Muscle Chow cooking. I use the butter spray when cooking eggs (see Chapter 7) and baking muffins or biscuits (see Chapter 11). Olive oil spray is perfect for pan cooking and for browning meats, plus you can mist a little on plain pasta or rice to add a light olive oil flavor. High-heat spray is excellent for coating a grill rack as well as metal skewers so food slides off easily. When I use cooking spray or olive oil to coat a skillet, I apply the spray or oil and then use a paper towel to wipe the inside of the skillet until it is only lightly coated. This helps cut needless fat from the meal while still maintaining a nonstick surface. Why use more oil than you absolutely have to?

☐ **Extra-virgin olive oil:** Olive oil has a 350°F smoke point, so it won't smoke or burn if kept to medium heat.

☐ **Oats**

☐ **Stevia:** Stevia is a plant that originated in Paraguay, with leaves that are 300 times sweeter than sugar (so it's all-natural instead of a man-made chemical). I've been using stevia powder as a sweetener for at least a decade now, and while it's becoming more popular, you'll be hard-pressed to find it in the sugar aisle at your grocery store. However, you can easily find it in just about any health food store—look near the herbal supplements for an array of products in both liquid and powder forms. I buy the individual 1-gram packets that come 50 or 100 per box. They travel easily, and there's no measuring involved. This all-natural sweetener is a great alternative to artificial sweeteners. It works just as well, dissolves quickly, contains no calories, and has little to no effect on blood sugar. I call for stevia in Muscle Chow recipes throughout this book. However, if you prefer a different sugar alternative, go ahead and substitute it.

☐ **Canned chicken:** Look for this in the same supermarket aisle where you find the canned tuna. I've tried most brands of canned chicken, and in my opinion Valley Fresh premium chunk chicken (in 3-ounce cans) is consistently the best one. In other brands, I've found pieces of bones and skin—a major yuck. The convenience of Valley Fresh's pop-top lid is also a plus. No can opener required. Just pop the top, but keep the lid on so you can drain and rinse the chicken twice to help reduce the sodium content.

☐ **Low-sodium canned tuna, packed in water**

☐ **Canned low-sodium sardines, packed in water**

☐ **Whey protein powder:** Using whey protein powder in a recipe can help balance the protein-to-carbohydrate ratio of a dish, thus allowing the body a more consistent glycemic response. This action helps our bodies run more efficiently by offering sustained energy and accentuating our fat-burning potential. Of the many protein powders on the market, I've found two that work great for many of the Muscle Chow recipes in this book: 100% Whey Gold Standard Protein and 100% Natural Whey Gold Standard by Optimum Nutrition. I'm not saying that this specific brand is the *only* one that you can or should use, but it's the one I've had very good success with. It can be found in health food stores everywhere.

- ☐ **Assorted pastas:** Recipes in Chapter 9 use rotini, ziti, linguine, small shells, lasagna, bow tie, and couscous.
- ☐ **No-salt canned tomato sauce**
- ☐ **Canned no-salt diced tomatoes**
- ☐ **Low-sodium pasta sauce**
- ☐ **Rice:** Recipes in Chapter 9 and elsewhere call for Arborio, basmati, wild, and quick-cooking varieties.
- ☐ **Plain couscous**
- ☐ **Assorted unsalted nuts:** Among the varieties used in Muscle Chow recipes are almonds (see Almond-Crusted Tilapia on page 116), walnuts (see Pear-Walnut Salad on page 176), and pecans (see Basic Granola Energy Mix on page 55).
- ☐ **All-natural peanut butter:** This type of peanut butter contains about $\frac{1}{4}$ cup of oil that separates and sits on the top. Smucker's Organic Chunky Peanut Butter is a brand that you'll find in any grocery store and is the one I use. Smucker's Natural Peanut Butter with Honey is pretty awesome too. When you first open the jar, pour off the oil and dump it into the trash. This will siphon off saturated fat. Then mix in 2 tablespoons of flaxseed oil and 1 tablespoon of whole flaxseeds. Now you've got healthy peanut butter spiked with essential fatty acids and extra fiber.
- ☐ **Applesauce:** Get the 4-ounce containers for convenient cooking and grab-and-go snacks.
- ☐ **Balsamic vinegar**
- ☐ **Dijon mustard**
- ☐ **Honey mustard**
- ☐ **Unsalted matzos**
- ☐ **Assorted no-salt canned beans:** Varieties specified in Muscle Chow recipes include kidney beans (see Muscle-Bound Chili on page 60), black soybeans (Baked Creamy Rice on page 148), and chickpeas (also called garbanzo beans, used in Tofu Bulgur Salad on page 150).
- ☐ **Low-sodium canned chicken and beef broth**
- ☐ **Canned fruit in water or light syrup**
- ☐ **4C® Carb Careful Plain Breadcrumbs:** I searched high and wide to find a basic breadcrumb mix suitable for the Muscle Chow kitchen and was more than pleased

to find these. They're made from soy flour and soy protein, so a single ⅓-cup serving packs an impressive 17 grams of protein and 5 grams of fiber, with only 9 grams of carbs and 5 milligrams of sodium. That makes them perfect for use in meatballs, meat loaf, and burgers, and as a breading for chicken or fish.

- ☐ **Bulgur wheat:** While this whole grain is best known for its role in tabbouleh, it can also be used in a number of other dishes, including baked goods, soups, and bean and vegetable burgers, to which it helps add bulk. On its own, bulgur can complement a variety of beef, fish, and poultry dishes. Nutritionally, bulgur wheat is high in fiber, so it helps lower cholesterol, regulates blood sugar levels to reduce insulin spikes, and makes you feel fuller for a longer period of time. One cup of bulgur wheat provides 24 grams of fiber—nearly the full daily recommended amount—plus 20 grams of protein, as much potassium as a banana (400 milligrams), and only 2 grams of fat.
- ☐ **Honey**
- ☐ **Brown sugar**
- ☐ **Hot-pepper sauce**
- ☐ **Worcestershire sauce**
- ☐ **Red wine vinegar**
- ☐ **Apple cider vinegar**
- ☐ **Whole wheat pastry flour**
- ☐ **Hain Pure Foods Featherweight Baking Powder:** As part of the Muscle Chow diet, I always try to cut excess sodium whenever possible, to help reduce water retention between the skin and muscle and look as cut as possible. While the average baking powder can add more than 400 milligrams of sodium per teaspoon, Hain Pure Foods Featherweight Baking Powder adds zero. That makes me feel warm and fuzzy on the inside—and look more ripped on the outside! You can find this baking powder at any health or whole foods market that carries baked goods, mixes, and spices. (I have even seen it at my local grocery store.)
- ☐ **Flaxseeds:** Whole flaxseeds can be stored in the pantry for up to a year until you're ready to grind them.
- ☐ **Low-fat graham crackers**
- ☐ **All-purpose flour**
- ☐ **No-sugar apple and cherry pie fillings**
- ☐ **Oat flour**
- ☐ **Oat bran**

- ☐ **Wheat bran**
- ☐ **Cornmeal**
- ☐ **Safflower oil:** With a smoke point of 460°F, safflower oil is good for cooking at higher temperatures.

HERBS AND SEASONINGS

- ☐ **Basil**
- ☐ **Oregano**
- ☐ **Parsley**
- ☐ **No-salt lemon-pepper seasoning**
- ☐ **McCormick Salt Free All-Purpose Seasoning:** This offers just the right blend of herbs and spices without adding any extra sodium to recipes. It consists of onion, parsley, basil, oregano, thyme, red pepper, garlic, lemon peel, celery, and paprika. Having all these flavors in one spice bottle is easy and convenient—two important requirements for the Muscle Chow kitchen. If you can't find this specific seasoning, check out McCormick Salt Free Garlic & Herb Seasoning. Or look for other brands that are sodium-free and boast similar herb and spice ingredients.
- ☐ **Chili powder**
- ☐ **Ground cinnamon**
- ☐ **Vanilla extract**
- ☐ **Ground black pepper**
- ☐ **Red-pepper flakes**
- ☐ **McCormick Imitation Butter Flavor:** This product is great in oatmeal, rice, and baked goods. I avoid powdered butter substitutes such as Molly McButter and Butter Buds because, while they are fat-free, they are high in sodium.
- ☐ **Ground red pepper**
- ☐ **Smoked paprika**
- ☐ **Minced garlic**
- ☐ **Rosemary**
- ☐ **Sage**
- ☐ **Thyme**
- ☐ **Nutmeg**
- ☐ **Cumin**
- ☐ **Allspice**
- ☐ **Sea salt**

TOOLS AND UTENSILS

- ☐ **Graduated measuring cups for dry ingredients**
- ☐ **Liquid measuring cups**
- ☐ **Measuring spoons**
- ☐ **All-purpose utility knife:** A good one that's slightly larger than a paring knife will be your go-to knife 90 percent of the time.
- ☐ **7-inch Santoku knife:** This is well-designed for chopping, with hollowed edges along the blade to keep foods from sticking.
- ☐ **Wooden spoons (with and without holes)**
- ☐ **Plastic spatula**
- ☐ **Tongs**
- ☐ **Mixing bowls**
- ☐ **Colander**
- ☐ **Large pot or saucepan with a lid**
- ☐ **Medium nonstick skillet with a glass lid**
- ☐ **Cutting board**
- ☐ **Potato masher**
- ☐ **Blender**
- ☐ **Whisk**
- ☐ **Grater**
- ☐ **Large roasting pan**
- ☐ **Large (3-quart) baking dish**
- ☐ **Nonstick loaf-size (9" × 5" × 3") baking pan**
- ☐ **Nonstick 12-cup muffin pan**
- ☐ **Plastic zip-top bags:** You can use these to divide everything you cook into single portions, to control your serving sizes and keep meals ready to transport and eat at any time. For example, in a single bag, I'll measure out about 15 baby carrots; 3 or 4 stalks of celery, halved; or 15 almonds. When I buy fresh ground meat, I make thin patties, individually wrap each one in plastic wrap, put them into a heavy-gauge zip-top bag, and throw them into the freezer. I do the same for chicken breasts, separating them into single-portion sizes with plastic wrap, then into a heavy-gauge zip-top bag and into the freezer. Of course, if I plan on chowing the meat within a few days, I store it in the fridge in the original package until I cook it. For convenience, it's always a good idea to cook enough for several days, then throw single portions of the cooked chicken breasts, beef, turkey, or fish into separate bags for on-the-go meals and snacks.

3

BREAKFAST

Even though you've been out of it for 8 hours, your body's been busy. Through the night, it's still humming along, repairing muscle fibers that you blitzed earlier that day.

Do the math: If you eat dinner at 7:00 p.m., hit the rack at 10:00 p.m., and wake up at 6:00 a.m., that's 11 hours without food. If you stretch your fast 'til a noontime lunch, you've basically starved your body for 17 hours. That leaves only 7 waking hours to provide an entire day's worth of nourishment. All that starvation time sends a signal to your body that hard times are at hand—and it promptly goes into fat-hoarding mode to see you through the perceived famine. That's why it's crucial that you feed your muscles first thing in the morning.

The solution is simple: Make time—even if it's only a few minutes—for breakfast. You can make some of the recipes in this chapter a day or two in advance for a grab-n-go morning snack. Try the granola recipes on pages 55 and 56. Want a hot meal? Each of the oatmeal recipes takes less than 4 minutes to whip up. And if you're looking for something to stick to your ribs, I've got you covered with blintzes and a selection of pancakes.

AVOCADO BREAKFAST

This meal packs a solid supply of healthy essential fatty acids (avocado, flaxseeds, and olive oil), so don't let the high fat content throw you off. EFAs are crucial for anyone interested in building muscle and staying lean. A diet lacking in these fats can lead to decreased production of hormones, including testosterone—a lack of which can cause decreased energy, vitality, libido, and muscle mass. Healthful fats also help your body use fat-soluble vitamins such as A, D, and E. The high fiber content of this dish is another plus. Munch on this breakfast and you can begin your day with a whopping 14 grams, which is nearly half the daily recommended fiber—probably close to what some people get in an entire day.

INGREDIENTS:

2	teaspoons honey mustard (use the lowest-sodium one you can find)
2	slices whole grain bread, toasted
½	avocado, peeled and sliced
½	tomato, thinly sliced
1	teaspoon extra-virgin olive oil
3	to 4 fresh basil leaves, chopped
½	tablespoon ground flaxseeds
	Ground black pepper

HOW TO MAKE IT:

STEP 1 Spread 1 teaspoon of the honey mustard on each piece of toast. Add half of the avocado and tomato to each slice. Drizzle each with the oil. Add half of the basil and flaxseeds. Sprinkle both with pepper (to taste).

STEP 2 After all the ingredients are loaded, I like to cut each piece of bread into quarters to make it easier to eat.

Makes 1 serving

Per serving: 394 calories, 11 g protein, 44 g carbohydrates, 21 g total fat, 2.5 g saturated fat, 14 g fiber, 112 mg sodium

VARIATIONS: Add a few thin slices of cucumber or a pinch of Parmesan cheese. If I've got fresh baby spinach handy in the fridge, I might add a few leaves between the avocado and the tomato.

MUFFAROONIES

INGREDIENTS:

1	English muffin, halved and toasted
4	thin slices fresh tomato
2	teaspoons flaxseed oil
1	teaspoon grated Parmesan cheese
4	fresh basil leaves
	Dash of ground black pepper

HOW TO MAKE IT:

STEP 1 Top each muffin half with 2 slices of tomato.

STEP 2 Drizzle with the oil.

STEP 3 Add the cheese.

STEP 4 Tear the basil into small pieces and sprinkle onto each Muffaroonie.

STEP 5 Season with the pepper.

Makes 1 serving

Per serving: 235 calories, 6 g protein, 29 g carbohydrates, 10.5 g total fat, 1.5 g saturated fat, 1 g fiber, 240 mg sodium

LEAN BLINTZES

INGREDIENTS:

FOR BATTER:

¾   **cup whole grain pastry flour**

1   **cup fat-free milk**

2   **egg whites**

⅛   **teaspoon Hain Pure Foods Featherweight Baking Powder**

FOR FILLING:

½   **cup fat-free ricotta cheese**

½   **cup low-fat, no-salt cottage cheese**

6   **tablespoons whole fruit blueberry preserves, or other fruit that you prefer**

HOW TO MAKE IT:

STEP 1 Combine the batter ingredients and mix well in a large bowl (it will be thin and runny).

STEP 2 Coat a nonstick skillet with cooking spray, then wipe away the excess with a paper towel and set aside the towel. Use this towel to lightly wipe the skillet between crepes. Heat the skillet over medium heat.

STEP 3 Pour in a small amount of batter (about ¼ cup), then tilt the pan to spread the batter to the edges, creating a thin crepe. (Using a thin layer of batter will ensure that you won't have to flip the crepe.)

STEP 4 Cook for 30 to 50 seconds, until the crepe begins to look dry and cooked through to the top. Carefully remove and set aside on a clean paper towel. Continue making the crepes, placing a paper towel between each one after cooking. Make 7 to 8 crepes, then pick the 6 best ones.

STEP 5 Preheat the oven to 350°F. Prepare the filling by mixing together the ricotta cheese and cottage cheese in a bowl.

STEP 6 Assemble the crepes: Lay a crepe on a plate, spoon 1 tablespoon of the filling in a line across the center of the crepe. Top with 1 tablespoon of the fruit preserves. Roll each crepe and place on nonstick foil.

STEP 7 Bake for 10 minutes, or just until the edges begin to brown.

Makes 3 servings

Per serving (2 blintzes): 260 calories, 16 g protein, 44 g carbohydrates, 1 g total fat, 0 g saturated fat, 5 g fiber, 144 mg sodium

LIGHT-AS-A-FEATHER BAKED GOODS

When it comes to baked goods, you want them light and fluffy. That's where baking powder comes in handy. When mixed with a liquid, baking powder reacts by producing little bubbles that help give baked goods more rise. In the end, you get fluffier pancakes, muffins, and breads. It's for this reason that recipes call for separating wet ingredients from dry ingredients. This way, when you mix the two together, the baking powder will react just before you cook the dish. I use Hain Pure Foods Featherweight Baking Powder, which is sodium-free.

MUSCLE TOAST

INGREDIENTS:

⅓   cup fat-free milk

2   large eggs

2   egg whites

2   scoops vanilla whey protein powder

½   teaspoon ground cinnamon

4   slices whole wheat bread

FRUIT TOPPING:

1   banana, mashed

1   tablespoon whole fruit strawberry
     preserves

1   tablespoon water

HOW TO MAKE IT:

STEP 1 Whisk together the milk, eggs, and egg whites in a large shallow bowl. Add the protein powder and cinnamon and whisk until completely mixed.

STEP 2 Soak the bread, one slice at a time, in the mixture for 30 seconds, or until soggy.

STEP 3 Coat a large skillet with cooking spray and heat over medium-high heat. Place the soaked bread in the skillet one or two slices at a time. Cook for 2 minutes, or until golden brown, then flip once and cook for 1 to 2 minutes longer, or until cooked through. The bread should be slightly firm to the touch.

STEP 4 While the bread is cooking, mix the banana, strawberry preserves, and water together in a bowl. Top each piece of toast with a spoonful of the topping.

Makes 2 servings

Per serving: 417 calories, 34 g protein, 57 g carbohydrates, 6 g total fat, 1.5 g saturated fat, 9 g fiber, 139 mg sodium

TOAST WITH WHOLE FRUIT PRESERVES

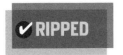

Some of us wake up and just aren't hungry first thing in the morning. Still, it's important to get something in your gut to jump-start your body's metabolism and your fat-burning potential for the day. Here's a simple breakfast that you just can't go wrong with. I'll chow this toast, then chug down a basic 90% Shake (see page 190) with my vitamins, and I'm good to go.

INGREDIENTS:

2   **slices whole grain bread**

1   **tablespoon any flavor of 100% whole fruit preserves**

1   **tablespoon ground flaxseeds**

HOW TO MAKE IT:

STEP 1 Toast the bread until crispy.

STEP 2 Spread the preserves over the toast.

STEP 3 Sprinkle with the flaxseeds, then cut the toast in half.

Makes 1 serving

Per serving: 250 calories, 11 g protein, 43 g carbohydrates, 4.5 g total fat, ½ g saturated fat, 10 g fiber, 5 mg sodium

RIPPED TIP

Serve a basic whey shake mixed with water to help increase the protein content of this meal. You can use the 90% Shake on page 190 if you'd like.

PROTEIN PANCAKES

Sneaking some protein powder into these pancakes helps make them

Muscle Chow–worthy. Unlike traditional pancakes (which are all

carbohydrates), these help you feel full while nourishing your muscles.

The recipes are simple—all you need for each are two bowls (one for

the dry ingredients, one for the wet) and a hot nonstick skillet or

griddle, then you're ready to build a stack. Serve your cakes with

sugar-free maple syrup, all-natural maple syrup, apple butter, or just

chow them plain.

BANANA PROTEIN PANCAKES

INGREDIENTS:

⅓   cup vanilla whey protein powder

⅓   cup whole grain pastry flour or all-purpose flour

¼   cup quick-cooking oats

1   packet (1 gram) stevia or other sugar alternative

1   teaspoon Hain Pure Foods Featherweight Baking Powder

1   banana, mashed

1   large egg

1   tablespoon fat-free plain yogurt

HOW TO MAKE IT:

STEP 1 In a large bowl, combine the protein powder, flour, oats, stevia, and baking powder. Mix well. Add the banana, egg, and yogurt. Mix.

STEP 2 Coat a nonstick skillet with cooking spray, then wipe away the excess with a paper towel and set aside the towel. Use this towel to wipe the skillet between pancakes, recoating the skillet with the oil and cleaning away any pancake batter crumbs. Heat the skillet over medium-low heat.

STEP 3 Spoon about ½ cup of the batter into the skillet. Cook for 1 to 2 minutes, or until firm and golden brown. Flip the pancake and cook for 30 seconds to 1 minute longer, or until golden brown. Remove the pancake to a plate. Wipe the skillet with the paper towel.

STEP 4 Repeat **STEP 3** with the remaining batter to make a total of 3 pancakes.

Makes 3 pancakes

Per pancake: 225 calories, 20 g protein, 27 g carbohydrates, 4 g total fat, 1 g saturated fat, 3 g fiber, 53 mg sodium

APPLE-WALNUT PROTEIN PANCAKES

INGREDIENTS:

1	cup quick-cooking oats
½	cup whole grain pastry flour
2	tablespoons chopped walnuts
1½	teaspoons Hain Pure Foods Featherweight Baking Powder
1	teaspoon ground cinnamon
1	scoop vanilla whey protein powder
3	egg whites
1	teaspoon pure vanilla extract
½	cup fat-free ricotta cheese
¾	cup fat-free milk

LEAN TIP

Linit yourself to 3 pancakes per sitting and store the rest in the fridge.

HOW TO MAKE IT:

STEP 1 Coat a nonstick skillet with cooking spray, then wipe away the excess with a paper towel and set aside the towel. Use this towel to wipe the skillet between pancakes, recoating the skillet with the oil and cleaning away any pancake batter crumbs. Preheat the skillet to medium-low, then reduce the heat to low.

STEP 2 Combine the dry ingredients in a bowl and mix well. Then add the wet ingredients and mix.

STEP 3 Spoon about ½ cup of the batter into the skillet. Cook for 1 to 2 minutes, or until firm and golden brown. Flip the pancake and finish cooking for 30 seconds to 1 minutes longer, or until golden brown. Remove the pancake to a plate. Wipe the skillet with the paper towel.

STEP 4 Repeat **STEP 3** with the remaining batter to make a total of 8 pancakes.

Makes 8 pancakes

Per pancake: 126 calories, 9 g protein, 16 g carbohydrates, 2 g total fat, 0 g saturated fat, 2 g fiber, 51 mg sodium

TIP It's important to cook pancakes over low heat to make sure they cook evenly. If the heat is too high, the outsides will burn while the insides remain runny.

ULTIMATE MUSCLE STACKS

The secret of this recipe's success is the specific ingredients it calls for.

☐ Friendship 1% Lowfat Cottage Cheese No Salt Added has the highest protein content (16 grams per ½ cup) and the lowest sodium (50 milligrams per ½ cup) of any cottage cheese that I've found. Since Friendship isn't a national brand, look for other low-sodium or no-salt cottage cheese brands in your local stores.

☐ There are two proteins to choose from for this recipe. EvoPro by CytoSport comes in several good-tasting flavors, including Berry Delicious and Tropical Blitz. It has 3 grams of L-glutamine, 23 grams of protein, and only 3 grams of carbohydrates per scoop. One container of this stuff will give you 16 batches of pancakes. Another good protein for this recipe is Lean Dessert Protein by BSN. It's available in an array of delicious varieties, including banana nut bread, fresh cinnamon roll, and whipped vanilla cream. Each scoop offers 20 grams of sustained-release protein, only 7 grams of carbs, plus digestive enzymes and no added aspartame or sugar.

INGREDIENTS:

1	cup unbleached or all-purpose flour
2	scoops (½ cup) CytoSport EvoPro protein powder or BSN Lean Dessert Protein powder
1½	teaspoons Hain Pure Foods Featherweight Baking Powder
2	large eggs
1	cup water
½	cup low-fat, no-salt cottage cheese
1	teaspoon McCormick Imitation Butter Flavor

HOW TO MAKE IT:

STEP 1 Coat a nonstick skillet with cooking spray, then wipe away the excess with a paper towel and set aside the towel. Use this towel to wipe the skillet between pancakes, recoating the skillet with the oil and cleaning away any pancake batter crumbs. Heat the skillet over medium-low heat.

STEP 2 In a bowl, combine the flour, protein powder, and baking powder. Mix well.

STEP 3 Add the eggs, water, cottage cheese, and butter flavor. Mix well.

STEP 4 Spoon about ½ cup of the batter into the skillet. Cook for 1 to 2 minutes, or until firm and golden brown. Flip the pancake and cook for 30 seconds to 1 minute longer, or until golden brown. Remove the pancake to a plate. Wipe the skillet with the paper towel.

STEP 5 Repeat Step 4 with the remaining batter to make a total of 8 pancakes.

Makes 8 pancakes

Per pancake: 123 calories, 11 g protein, 14 g carbohydrates, 2 g total fat, ½ g saturated fat, ½ g fiber, 37 mg sodium

OATS: THE CHAMPION OF LOW-GLYCEMIC CARBS

Look at any nutrition publication and you'll find that oats are

consistently ranked among the top-10 best foods that you can chow.

Whether you buy old-fashioned rolled oats, quick-cooking rolled oats,

or hearty steel-cut oats, they're all easy to prepare in just minutes. (I

use old-fashioned oats most of the time because they're less

processed than the quick-cooking, which means they're less

glycemic—they won't spike insulin levels and cause you to store fat.)

One thing's for certain, oats have a great taste and texture. You can

chow them cooked or raw and add them to recipes easily. Because

oats are high in fiber, they are digested more slowly and make you feel

fuller longer. They're probably best known for helping lower cholesterol

levels, a benefit that's stamped on just about every container and backed by the American Heart Association. They're also high in

minerals like magnesium for energy production, iron for blood support,

manganese to help with blood sugar regulation, and selenium to help

support thyroid function and its role in regulating fat metabolism. As

an added benefit for us muscleheads, oats are also relatively high in

protein, yielding approximately 5 grams per half cup. The bottom line

is that oats should be a part of everyone's diet, and they play a

significant role in the Muscle Chow diet.

PROTEIN OATS

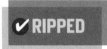
✔ RIPPED

INGREDIENTS:

1	cup water
¾	cup oats
1½	scoops whey protein powder
½	cup fat-free milk
1	packet (1 gram) stevia or other sugar alternative
1	teaspoon ground cinnamon
1	banana, sliced (optional)

HOW TO MAKE IT:

STEP 1 In a microwaveable bowl, combine the water and oats. Microwave on high for 3½ minutes.

STEP 2 In a shaker bottle, combine the protein powder and milk. Shake to mix.

STEP 3 When the oats are ready, add the stevia and cinnamon. Stir to mix. Add the protein shake and stir again until mixed and smooth.

STEP 4 Add the sliced banana on top, or chow plain.

Makes 1 serving

Per serving: 478 calories, 48 g protein, 60 g carbohydrates, 7 g total fat, 1 g saturated fat, 8 g fiber, 117 mg sodium

VARIATION: Instead of using vanilla whey protein all the time (which is good), I also like to use banana- or strawberry-flavored whey protein to help punch up the taste. If you make this substitution, omit the cinnamon because it doesn't go with those flavors very well. The next time you're at the health food store, get creative and look for different flavored proteins. For other protein flavor ideas, check out Ultimate Muscle Stacks on page 47.

RIPPED TIP
Use ½ cup water in place of the milk.

HEARTY OATMEAL 'N' BRAN

INGREDIENTS:

1½	cups water
⅓	cup plus 1 tablespoon oats
2	packets (2 grams) stevia or other sugar alternative
¼	teaspoon McCormick Imitation Butter Flavor
⅓	cup oat bran
1	tablespoon chopped mixed nuts (almonds, walnuts, cashews, etc.)
1	tablespoon raisins
¼	cup fat-free milk
1	banana, sliced (optional)

HOW TO MAKE IT:

STEP 1 In a microwaveable bowl, combine the water, oats, stevia, and butter flavor. Microwave on high for 3½ minutes.

STEP 2 Add the oat bran, nuts, raisins, milk, and banana (if using). Stir well and enjoy.

Makes 1 serving

Per serving: 311 calories, 14 g protein, 57 g carbohydrates, 9 g total fat, 1 g saturated fat, 10 g fiber, 88 mg sodium

APPLES 'N' OATS

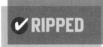

INGREDIENTS:

1	apple, peeled and chopped
1½	cups water
½	cup Quaker Oat Bran Hot Cereal
1	tablespoon raisins
½	teaspoon ground cinnamon
¼	teaspoon pure vanilla extract
1	packet (1 gram) stevia or other sugar alternative

HOW TO MAKE IT:

STEP 1 In a microwaveable bowl, combine the apple, water, and cereal. Microwave on high for 3 minutes.

STEP 2 Add the raisins, cinnamon, vanilla extract, and stevia. Mix well.

Makes 1 serving

Per serving: 179 calories, 3 g protein, 42 g carbohydrates, 1.5 g total fat, 0 g saturated fat, 5 g fiber, 93 mg sodium

RIPPED TIP

Add a basic whey shake such as the 90% Shake on page 190 to help increase the protein content of this meal.

OAT PEACHES 'N' CREAM

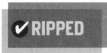

INGREDIENTS:

1¼	**cups water**
½	**cup Quaker Oat Bran Hot Cereal**
¼	**teaspoon McCormick Imitation Butter Flavor**
1	**scoop vanilla whey protein powder**
½	**cup fat-free milk**
1	**peach, pitted and cut into thin wedges**
1	**packet (1 gram) stevia or other sugar alternative**

HOW TO MAKE IT:

STEP 1 In a microwaveable bowl, combine the water, cereal, and butter flavor. Microwave on high for 3 minutes.

STEP 2 In a shaker bottle, combine the protein powder and milk. Shake to mix.

STEP 3 Pour the protein shake into the cooked oats a little at a time, stopping to mix, until the consistency is thick and not runny. Drink any of the shake that's left over.

STEP 4 Add the peach wedges and stevia and mix.

Makes 1 serving

Per serving: 296 calories, 31 g protein, 42 g carbohydrates, 2 g total fat, 1 g saturated fat, 4 g fiber, 186 mg sodium

RIPPED TIP
Use ½ cup water in place of the milk.

OATMEAL WITH FRUIT AND NUTS

INGREDIENTS:

1½	cups water
¾	cup oats
5	almonds, crushed
1	tablespoon raisins (optional)
1	packet (1 gram) stevia or other sugar alternative
¼	teaspoon pure vanilla extract
	Pinch of ground cinnamon
½	banana, sliced

HOW TO MAKE IT:

STEP 1 In a microwaveable bowl, combine the water and oats. Microwave on high for 3½ minutes.

STEP 2 Add the almonds, raisins (if using), stevia, vanilla extract, and cinnamon. Mix well.

STEP 3 Top with the banana and enjoy.

Makes 1 serving

Per serving: 359 calories, 10 g protein, 61 g carbohydrates, 5 g total fat, 0 g saturated fat, 10 g fiber, 10 mg sodium

BASIC GRANOLA ENERGY MIX

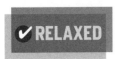
✔ RELAXED

INGREDIENTS:

2½	cups oats
½	cup unsalted roasted almonds
½	cup pecans
½	cup toasted wheat germ
½	cup (or 1 4-ounce container) unsweetened applesauce
¼	cup warm water
3	tablespoons whole flaxseeds
2	tablespoons brown sugar
1	tablespoon molasses
½	teaspoon ground cinnamon
½	teaspoon pure vanilla extract
¼	teaspoon ground nutmeg
¼	cup dried pineapple chunks
¼	cup dried cherries
2	tablespoons shredded coconut

TIP Store in an airtight container to ensure freshness.

HOW TO MAKE IT:

STEP 1 Preheat the oven to 350°F.

STEP 2 In a large bowl, mix together all the ingredients except the pineapple, cherries, and coconut.

STEP 3 Coat a large baking pan with cooking spray. Add the mixture and spread it from edge to edge to create an even layer.

STEP 4 Bake for 90 minutes, stirring every 15 minutes, until all the granola is browned and crunchy.

STEP 5 Remove from the oven and allow it to cool completely.

STEP 6 Add the pineapple, cherries, and coconut. Stir to mix.

Makes 7 servings

Per serving (½ cup): 351 calories, 11 g protein, 44 g carbohydrates, 16 g total fat, 1.5 g saturated fat, 9 g fiber, 7 mg sodium

VARIATION: You could substitute 1 tablespoon raisins, 3 tablespoons chopped dates, and/or ¼ cup dried strawberries for any or all of the dried fruits (coconut, pineapple, or cherries) in this recipe.

PROTEIN GRANOLA

Heart-healthy oatmeal with nuts and raisins is one of my favorite breakfasts. It's a cholesterol- and sodium-free food that's also high in fiber, so it makes you feel full and ready to start the day. Because oats are a low-glycemic carb, you can have them at any time of the day. Protein Granola takes oatmeal to the next level. I've added all kinds of goodness—almonds, flaxseeds, wheat germ, whey protein, and more—to create a granola cereal that's loaded with all the ingredients made for an active lifestyle. Pour some in a bowl and eat it with fat-free milk, or take it on the run and munch it dry. It makes a great snack. Either way, I guarantee it won't last long. The bottom line is that you'll have a hard time finding another granola cereal that boasts the nutritional profile of this one.

INGREDIENTS:

3	cups oats
½	cup unsalted roasted almonds
3	tablespoons whole flaxseeds
1	teaspoon ground cinnamon
1	cup toasted wheat germ
4	scoops vanilla whey protein powder
2	tablespoons brown sugar
3	tablespoons honey
1	cup water
3	tablespoons dried cranberries
3	tablespoons chopped dates
2	tablespoons raisins

HOW TO MAKE IT:

STEP 1 Preheat the oven to 350°F.

STEP 2 In a large bowl, mix together all the ingredients except the cranberries, dates, and raisins.

STEP 3 Coat a large baking pan with cooking spray. Add the mixture and spread from edge to edge to create an even layer.

STEP 4 Bake for 90 minutes, stirring every 15 minutes, until all the granola is browned and crunchy. If it's not crunchy after 90 minutes, bake for 15 minutes longer while watching to see that it doesn't get too dark.

STEP 5 Remove from the oven and allow it to cool completely.

STEP 6 Add the cranberries, dates, and raisins. Stir to mix.

Makes 7 servings

Per serving (½ cup): 418 calories, 23 g protein, 58 g carbohydrates, 12 g total fat, 1 g saturated fat, 9 g fiber, 26 mg sodium

TIP Separate ½-cup portions into individual baggies so you don't overeat in one sitting. Store them in an airtight container.

4

BEEF

Beef is a great source of muscle-building protein, with 6 ounces of meat yielding 36 grams of protein. It contains a complete spectrum of amino acids as well as natural creatine to help repair muscle tissue and increase size and strength. It's high in iron for healthy blood, vitamin B12 for energy production, zinc for hormone health and immune function, plus selenium and glutathione, two antioxidants for cellular health.

One of the by-products of intense training is the formation of free radicals. When you're on those last couple of reps and you feel your muscles burning, that sensation is lactic acid buildup. The next day, you might experience muscle soreness due to muscle fiber breakdown (delayed onset muscle soreness, or DOMS). In turn, this triggers an increase in blood flow to those muscles to help facilitate recovery and repair by transporting amino acids to muscle cells. The blood flow also helps shuttle powerful antioxidants like selenium and glutathione throughout the body to help neutralize free radicals. Eating meat can be a good way to ensure you get the crucial antioxidants needed to fight those free radicals.

What about the fat? Sure, beef contains fat, and that's why it's important to choose the leanest cuts (see "Buy the Best" on page 58). Lots of people tend to go for marbled beef that's higher in saturated fat, because it's supposed to be juicier and better tasting. Not us—we're modern-day gladiators whose goal is to feed our bodies the right

BUY THE BEST

Read package labels. Eighty percent lean also means that beef is 20 percent fat. Look for "extra lean" or "select"—those meats contain the least amount of fat (15 percent or less). And while these are said to be less juicy and less tender than marbled beef, I believe they're just as good so long as you don't overcook them. Ground beef is my favorite choice for tender, juicy, flavorful meat, and I look for 95 percent lean or less. No matter what cuts of beef you choose, when making your selections, be sure to look for a nice red color without a lot of marbling. If it looks good and feels tender, it probably is. Some of the leanest cuts—such as tenderloin, eye of round, top loin, sirloin tip, and bottom round— yield as little as 6 grams of fat per 6 ounces, with a solid 36 grams of muscle-building protein.

foods to promote muscle repair and growth (i.e., Muscle Chow) and build athletic performance and a physique that's esthetically pleasing. Lean cuts of beef offer just the right amount of saturated fat to fuel your body's testosterone production. That's probably the biggest reason I crave a really good burger, because most all of the saturated fat that I get in my diet usually comes from two food sources: beef and eggs. I can feel the power surge through my veins when I digest these kinds of foods. Bottom line: Beef is a catalyst that can help raise testosterone levels as well as pack on muscle mass.

HORMONE-FREE, CAGE-FREE, GRASS-FED MEATS

Today, every health food market and even the average grocery store carries lean beef, pork, and chicken that has been produced without antibiotics, pesticides, and steroids, chemicals that, when consumed over time, can tax your endocrine system and interfere with the natural balance of your hormones. This, plus the ways in which animals are treated, are two important factors for me. Even though an animal might be hormone-free, that doesn't necessarily mean it's also free to roam and graze in its natural setting. Research shows that cage-free chickens produce eggs much higher in omega-3s than those laid by their cooped-up counterparts. And free-roaming cows chowing on pasture grass offer as much as four times more vitamin E and conjugated linoleic acid than cattle penned up in tight quarters. (Conjugated linoleic acid—also known as CLA—is a fat that helps enhance muscle growth and reduce body fat.) Nutritionally, free-roaming grass-fed animals are superior due to the nutrients that naturally occur in the grass and insects they consume.

POWER BURGER

On those days when you've had an especially tough workout, this is all you need to feed your hungry muscles. This burger offers solid protein to repair tissue; iron and vitamin B12 to restore energy; and added ingredients that offer an array of B vitamins, calcium, magnesium, vitamin E, and antioxidants.

INGREDIENTS:

1	**pound extra-lean ground beef**
1	**tablespoon sunflower seeds**
1	**tablespoon finely chopped onion**
1	**tablespoon finely chopped red bell pepper**
¼	**teaspoon ground black pepper**
1	**cup toasted wheat germ**
4	**whole grain burger buns**
	Lettuce (optional)
	Tomato, thinly sliced (optional)
	Honey mustard (optional)

HOW TO MAKE IT:

STEP 1 Preheat a grill or skillet to medium-low.

STEP 2 Place the ground beef in a large mixing bowl, and add all the ingredients except the wheat germ and buns. Knead with your hands until everything is well mixed.

STEP 3 Form into 4 patties. Roll the patties in the wheat germ until they're covered.

STEP 4 Grill or pan-fry for 8 to 10 minutes for medium or 14 to 18 minutes for well-done.

STEP 5 Place each burger on a bun. Top with the lettuce, tomato, and mustard (if using).

Makes 4 servings

Per serving: 367 calories, 35 g protein, 37 g carbohydrates, 11 g total fat, 2.5 g saturated fat, 8 g fiber, 272 mg sodium

SERVING SUGGESTION: Serve with apple wedges to help pump up the total carbs, especially when eating this as a postworkout glycogen-replenishing meal.

TIP Buy 2 pounds of ground beef and double the recipe. Freeze any extra burgers for later. Form the patties, wrap them individually in plastic wrap, then put them in a heavy-duty zip-top bag to avoid freezer burn. Before you hit the gym, take one out and throw it into the fridge. By the time you get home, it will be thawed and ready to cook.

MUSCLE-BOUND CHILI

INGREDIENTS:

2	pounds extra-lean ground beef
½	teaspoon ground black pepper
2	medium sweet onions, finely chopped
1	tablespoon chopped garlic
2	cans (14–15 ounces each) no-salt diced tomatoes
1	can (15 ounces) no-salt kidney beans, rinsed and drained
1	can (6 ounces) unsalted tomato paste
½	cup water
¼	cup red wine (such as cabernet sauvignon)
2	tablespoons chili powder
½	teaspoon ground red pepper
½	teaspoon smoked paprika
½	teaspoon ground cumin

HOW TO MAKE IT:

STEP 1 In a large skillet, combine the ground beef and black pepper. Cook over medium-high heat for 4 minutes, or until no longer pink. Drain and set aside.

STEP 2 In a large pot, combine the onions and garlic. Cook on medium-high heat for 2 to 3 minutes, or until the onions are translucent.

STEP 3 Add the ground beef and the rest of the ingredients to the pot. Bring to a boil, stirring occasionally. Reduce the heat to low, cover the pot, and simmer for 30 minutes, stirring occasionally.

Makes 8 servings

Per serving: 224 calories, 26 g protein, 17 g carbohydrates, 5 g total fat, 1.5 g saturated fat, 4 g fiber, 130 mg sodium

BEEFCAKE MEAT LOAF

INGREDIENTS:

1	pound extra-lean ground beef
2	egg whites
1	zucchini, coarsely grated
1	rib celery, finely chopped
½	small yellow onion, finely chopped
½	cup quick-cooking oats
¼	cup toasted wheat germ
2	tablespoons sliced black olives
1	teaspoon dried oregano
¼	teaspoon ground black pepper
1	cup no-salt tomato sauce

HOW TO MAKE IT:

STEP 1 Preheat the oven to 350°F. Coat a nonstick 9" × 5" loaf pan with cooking spray. Wipe away any excess with a paper towel.

STEP 2 Place all of the ingredients except for the tomato sauce in a large bowl. Add ¼ cup of the tomato sauce and reserve the rest. Use your hands to mix everything together well.

STEP 3 Place the meat mixture into the pan and shape from edge to edge so it's even. Pour the remaining ¾ cup tomato sauce over the top.

STEP 4 Bake for 50 minutes, or until a thermometer inserted in the center registers 160°F and the meat is no longer pink. Remove the pan to a rack and let the meatloaf sit for about 10 minutes before removing from the pan and slicing.

Makes 4 servings

Per serving: 249 calories, 29 g protein, 19 g carbohydrates, 6.5 g total fat, 2 g saturated fat, 4 g fiber, 137 mg sodium

MEATHEAD TACO SALAD

Quick and easy, nutritious and refreshing—make it once and you'll be addicted to this salad.

INGREDIENTS:

½	pound extra-lean ground beef
2	teaspoons chili powder
3	drops of hot-pepper sauce
	Pinch of ground black pepper
2	cups shredded iceberg lettuce
1	tomato, finely chopped
2	tablespoons shredded low-fat Cheddar cheese

HOW TO MAKE IT:

STEP 1 Lightly coat a large nonstick skillet with cooking spray. Wipe away any excess with a paper towel. Heat the skillet to medium.

STEP 2 Add the ground beef and break it apart with a wooden spoon as it's heating up. Add the chili powder, hot-pepper sauce, and black pepper. Cook for 6 to 8 minutes, or until no longer pink. Drain and set aside.

STEP 3 In a large single-serving bowl, layer the lettuce, beef mixture, tomato, and cheese.

Makes 1 serving

Per serving: 332 calories, 50 g protein, 10 g carbohydrates, 10.5 g total fat, 3.5 g saturated fat, 3 g fiber, 268 mg sodium

SERVING SUGGESTION: The salad is awesome just like this, but for added punch you can add half of an avocado, diced, and/or a couple tablespoons of low-sodium salsa.

BEEF BOMBS

INGREDIENTS:

4	bell peppers (green, yellow, or red)
¼	teaspoon extra-virgin olive oil
1	pound extra-lean ground beef
1	egg white
½	cup finely chopped yellow onion
2	tablespoons no-salt canned corn
1	tablespoon finely chopped dried or fresh parsley
¼	cup toasted wheat germ
	Pinch of ground black pepper
¾	cup low-sodium tomato or spaghetti sauce
1	teaspoon prepared horseradish

HOW TO MAKE IT:

STEP 1 Preheat the oven to 425°F. Pour ¼" of water into a baking pan. Cut off the tops of the bell peppers, then carefully remove the seeds and membranes (pinch them out with your fingers or use a paring knife) and discard. Lightly coat the skins of the peppers with the oil. Place the peppers cut side down into the baking pan. Bake for 10 minutes.

STEP 2 In a large bowl, mix together the beef, egg white, onion, corn, parsley, wheat germ, black pepper, and ¼ cup of the sauce.

STEP 3 When the peppers are ready, remove them from the oven. Reduce the heat to 350°F. Fill each pepper with ¼ of the beef mixture, then return the peppers to the baking pan cut side up (the pan should still have about ¼" of water in it).

STEP 4 Bake for 30 minutes. Stir together the horseradish and the remaining ½ cup tomato sauce and add a little to the top of each pepper. Bake for 15 minutes longer, or until the meat is no longer pink.

Makes 4 servings

Per serving: 217 calories, 27 g protein, 16 g carbohydrates, 6 g total fat, 2 g saturated fat, 4 g fiber, 96 mg sodium

TIP You can refrigerate any leftover Beef Bombs for up to 2 days. Then either chow them cold, heat them up in a toaster oven at 350°F for 15 to 20 minutes, or throw them in the microwave for a few minutes. They make a quick and satisfying meal anytime.

GRILLED TENDERLOIN STEAK

INGREDIENTS:

2	lean beef tenderloin steaks (each 5 to 6 ounces and about 1" thick)
½	teaspoon + 1 dash ground black pepper
10	large asparagus spears, with tough ends cut off
1	large tomato, sliced into ¾"-thick rounds
½	teaspoon no-salt lemon-pepper seasoning

HOW TO MAKE IT:

STEP 1 Trim any fatty edges from the steaks. Sprinkle the ½ teaspoon black pepper onto both sides and gently rub into the steaks. Set aside.

STEP 2 Coat a grill rack with high-heat cooking spray. Preheat the grill to medium.

STEP 3 Lightly coat the asparagus and tomato with olive oil cooking spray. Sprinkle the lemon-pepper seasoning on the asparagus and the dash black pepper on the tomatoes.

STEP 4 For medium doneness, grill the steaks for 3 to 4 minutes on each side, or until a thermometer inserted in the center registers 160°F. For medium-well doneness, grill the steaks for 5 to 6 minutes per side, or until a thermometer inserted in the center registers 165°F. The steaks should be lightly charred on the outside and slightly pink in the center for perfect juicy tenderness.

STEP 5 Just before you turn the steaks, add the asparagus and tomatoes to the grill rack (be sure to lay the asparagus horizontally so the spears don't fall through the grate). Grill the veggies for 3 to 4 minutes on each side, or until slightly charred.

Makes 2 servings

Per serving: 188 calories, 31 g protein, 8 g carbohydrates, 5 g total fat, 2 g saturated fat, 3 g fiber, 73 mg sodium

SERVING SUGGESTION: Serve with a cup of plain wild rice to help balance the carbs-to-protein ratio. Cook the rice according to the package directions, but be sure to leave out any salt, butter, or oil. To give the rice a buttery flavor, use a little fat-free pump-spray butter (which you can find in the dairy section of any grocery store).

LONDON BROIL

INGREDIENTS:

1½	pounds lean top round roast, trimmed of fat
½	cup balsamic vinegar
2	tablespoons brown sugar
1	tablespoon extra-virgin olive oil
1	teaspoon Worcestershire sauce
½	teaspoon chopped dried or fresh parsley
¼	teaspoon ground black pepper
¼	teaspoon onion powder

HOW TO MAKE IT:

STEP 1 Use a sharp knife to score the roast diagonally about ¼" deep. Cut again in the opposite direction to create diamond scores. Do this on both sides of the roast.

STEP 2 In a large zip-top bag, combine the rest of the ingredients. Add the beef and seal the bag. Marinate in the fridge for at least 6 hours (overnight is even better).

STEP 3 Adjust the oven rack to the highest level. Preheat the broiler.

STEP 4 Place the roast on a broiler pan. Discard the marinade. Broil the roast for 6 minutes on each side, or until a thermometer inserted in the center registers 160°F for medium doneness. The outside should be crusty and sizzling and the inside slightly pink.

STEP 5 Remove from the oven and transfer to a cutting board. Tent with foil and allow the roast to rest for 10 minutes before slicing. This makes for a juicier London broil.

STEP 6 Make very thin slices diagonally across the grain.

Makes 5 servings

Per serving: 255 calories, 29 g protein, 9 g carbohydrates, 10 g total fat, 3 g saturated fat, 0 g fiber, 96 mg sodium

SERVING SUGGESTION: Serve with a side of orzo pasta and steamed veggies to help balance out the carbs-to-protein ratio. Orzo is a type of pasta that looks similar to rice. Cook it according to the package directions, then finish it off by adding a teaspoon of extra-virgin olive oil and some chopped parsley.

TIP While broiling, crack the oven door slightly (about an inch). This will keep the oven coils activated and red hot, preventing them from cycling off. This beef is just as tasty when cooked on the grill. Preheat the grill to medium-high and grill the roast for 6 to 7 minutes on each side.

FILET WITH ROASTED CARROTS

Filet mignon on the grill is tasty and tender, without greasy saturated fat. Because it's cut from the loin, it is naturally lean. New York strip is another good lean option. For the best of both worlds, pick up a porterhouse steak. This cut includes both the New York strip and the filet mignon. I don't like to add a bunch of spices that mask the flavor of the beef—I prefer to keep it simple, flavoring with just olive oil and ground black pepper.

Heirloom (or rainbow) carrots aren't always easy to find, but they're well worth the hunt. Orange heirlooms are a staple at healthy food markets; while you're there, look for yellow, red, and even purple heirloom carrots as well. Colors like these indicate that the carrot pigments contain antioxidants such as lycopene (also found in tomatoes and berries) and especially beta-carotene (also in sweet potatoes and squash). These antioxidants offer health benefits such as immune support, tissue growth and repair, and hormone balance. If you can't find heirlooms, just substitute regular small carrots that come bunched together with the stems still attached (like Bugs Bunny might chow).

INGREDIENTS:

4   filets mignons (each 6 to 8 ounces and 1¼" to 1½" thick)

2   pounds small heirloom carrots

        Pinch of sea salt

2   teaspoons extra-virgin olive oil

        Ground black pepper

4   pitas or lavash (choose the lowest fat and sodium brand you can find)

1   bunch fresh parsley, chopped

HOW TO MAKE IT:

STEP 1   Preheat the grill to high. Trim the filets of any excess fat, then let them sit at room temperature for about 20 minutes while you prepare the carrots.

STEP 2   Preheat the oven to 400°F. Trim the leaves from the carrots, leaving ¼" of the stems. Wash the carrots.

WHAT'S LAVASH?

Lavash is thin flat bread made with a few basic ingredients: wheat flour, water, and yeast. You can find it in the bakery section of any healthy food store. I like it because it's simple, low-sodium, and made without a bunch of added ingredients. Do I eat it all the time? No—but it's nice to have every once in a while.

STEP 3 Coat a 12" × 9" baking pan with cooking spray. Wipe away any excess with a paper towel. Add the carrots and sprinkle with the salt. Add 1 teaspoon of the oil and toss until the carrots are well coated with oil. Set aside.

STEP 4 Pat the filets with a paper towel, then brush with the remaining 1 teaspoon oil. Rub pepper (to taste) on both sides of each filet.

STEP 5 On the grill, sear the filets for 2 minutes on each side, to seal in the juices and flavor. Reduce the heat to medium. For medium-rare filets, grill for 10 to 12 minutes longer, or until a thermometer inserted in the center registers 145°F, turning once or twice. For medium filets, grill for 15 to 20 minutes, or until a thermometer registers 160°F.

STEP 6 While the filets are grilling, bake the carrots for 12 to 15 minutes, stirring once halfway to ensure even cooking.

STEP 7 Just before the filets are done, put the pitas or lavash on the grill for 1 minute to lightly toast.

STEP 8 Serve the filets with the roasted carrots and warm pitas or lavash on the side. Garnish the plates by sprinkling a little parsley over each.

Makes 4 servings

Per serving: 327 calories, 37 g protein, 28 g carbohydrates, 8 g total fat, 2.5 g saturated fat, 8 g fiber, 281 mg sodium

TIP Most people would tell you to look for well-marbled beef because it has more flavor, but marbling just means more fat. I recommend looking for beef that's bright red and just lightly marbled. Remember, this is food with a function, and there's still plenty of good flavor in a nice lean filet.

PALOMILLA PEPPER STEAK

INGREDIENTS:

1	teaspoon extra-virgin olive oil
1	medium green bell pepper, sliced into ½" strips
½	cup chopped sweet onion
¼	teaspoon ground black pepper
20	grape tomatoes (or 10 cherry tomatoes cut in half)
1	pound top sirloin steak, sliced into ½"-wide strips
½	teaspoon Worcestershire sauce
	Red-pepper flakes
1	tablespoon lime juice (about half a lime)

HOW TO MAKE IT:

STEP 1 In a large skillet over medium-high heat, combine the oil, green pepper, onion, and black pepper. Cook, stirring frequently, for 5 minutes, or until the onion becomes translucent.

STEP 2 Add the tomatoes and cook, stirring frequently, for 1 minute.

STEP 3 Add the steak, Worcestershire sauce, and red-pepper flakes (to taste). Cook, stirring frequently, for 3 to 4 minutes, or until the steak strips are browned at the edges but slightly pink in the middle, for medium doneness.

STEP 4 Add the lime juice and remove the meal to 2 plates.

Makes 2 servings

Per serving: 374 calories, 51 g protein, 11 g carbohydrates, 13 g total fat, 4 g saturated fat, 3 g fiber, 151 mg sodium

MAKE IT BETTER WITH BUFFALO

You've probably heard that buffalo is leaner than beef, and it is. In fact,

pound for pound, lean cuts of buffalo have less fat than chicken. Plus,

buffalo aren't subject to hormones and other growth stimulants like

beef and poultry are. If you've ever seen one in person, you know that

they're huge animals—and that's without any added hormones. I like

the flavor almost as much as that of regular lean beef, and buffalo

meat isn't difficult to find nowadays. You can usually get ground

buffalo at your local grocery store. If not, health food markets that

carry fresh meats will have it for sure.

SIMPLE BUFFALO BURGERS

INGREDIENTS:

1	pound lean ground buffalo
¼	cup finely chopped onion
1	tablespoon chopped dried or fresh parsley
½	teaspoon Worcestershire sauce
¼	teaspoon ground black pepper
4	whole grain burger buns

HOW TO MAKE IT:

STEP 1 Preheat the grill to medium.

STEP 2 Place all the ingredients except the buns in a large mixing bowl and knead with your hands until mixed well.

STEP 3 Form into 4 patties about ½" thick so they cook fast.

STEP 4 Grill for 8 minutes per side, or until a thermometer inserted in the center registers 160°F and the meat is no longer pink.

STEP 5 Slide each burger onto a bun.

Makes 4 servings

Per serving: 259 calories, 28 g protein, 23 g carbohydrates, 6 g total fat, 2 g saturated fat, 3 g fiber, 263 mg sodium

SERVING SUGGESTION: Top with lettuce, tomato, onion, and Dijon mustard. Serve with On-the-Go Cottage Cheese 'n' Bananas on page 217.)

TIP These freeze just as well as regular beef burgers. Wrap each patty in plastic wrap, then store them in a heavy-duty zip-top bag to avoid freezer burn. When you're in the mood for a buffalo burger, just pull one out in the morning and throw it in the fridge to thaw for later.

BAKED BISON MEATBALLS

INGREDIENTS:

1	pound lean ground buffalo
2	egg whites
½	cup toasted wheat germ
⅓	cup finely chopped onion
1	tablespoon grated Parmesan cheese
1	teaspoon jarred minced garlic
½	teaspoon McCormick Salt Free All-Purpose Seasoning
¼	teaspoon ground black pepper

HOW TO MAKE IT:

STEP 1 Preheat the oven to 400°F. Lightly coat a baking pan with cooking spray. Wipe away any excess with a paper towel.

STEP 2 Put all the ingredients in a large mixing bowl and knead with your hands until everything is mixed well.

STEP 3 Shape into approximately 20 golf ball–size meatballs and place them on the baking pan.

STEP 4 Bake for 15 minutes, turning once after 7 minutes, or until no longer pink.

Makes 4 servings

Per serving: 218 calories, 31 g protein, 9 g carbohydrates, 6 g total fat, 2 g saturated fat, 2 g fiber, 98 mg sodium

SERVING SUGGESTION: Place 5 meatballs and 1 cup low-sodium tomato sauce (per person) in a saucepan and warm over medium heat until the sauce begins to bubble. Gently stir for 3 to 5 minutes, or until the sauce is heated through. Serve over spaghetti.

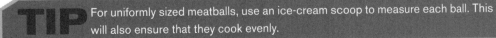

TIP For uniformly sized meatballs, use an ice-cream scoop to measure each ball. This will also ensure that they cook evenly.

5

CHICKEN

Chicken has to be one of the most widely eaten animal proteins on the planet. It's relatively inexpensive, super lean, and packed with protein, and it can be prepared a slew of different ways. It's a great alternative to red meat because it has a fraction of the fat, thus allowing you to stay lean while still ensuring that your body has enough protein for muscle synthesis. A single chicken breast contains 25 to 30 grams of protein, no carbs, and less than 2 grams of fat. With a nutritional profile like that, it makes sense to cook several pieces at a time and store them in the fridge for a quick on-the-go meal. In fact, throw them into separate zip-top baggies so you don't waste time, then grab an apple, and you've got my version of fast food. When you're eating out in restaurants, you'll rarely have trouble finding chicken on the menu, and it can easily be ordered grilled plain with a side of steamed veggies or topped over a salad.

2-MINUTE CHICKEN SALAD PITA

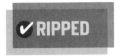 **✔ RIPPED**

In just three easy steps, you can whip up one of the best-tasting chicken salad sandwiches ever. When I'm in a hurry and only have a couple of minutes (literally), this makes for a great meal. Just keep these simple ingredients on hand, and it's a snap—2 minutes from start to finish.

INGREDIENTS:

1   pita (choose the lowest fat and sodium brand you can find)

1   can (3 ounces) chunk chicken, rinsed and drained twice

1   teaspoon fat-free sour cream

1   teaspoon fat-free plain yogurt

1   teaspoon spicy brown mustard

Pinch of McCormick Salt Free It's a Dilly Seasoning, or equal parts dried dill and ground black pepper

½   cup shredded lettuce

HOW TO MAKE IT:

STEP 1   Put the pita in the toaster oven and lightly toast to warm.

STEP 2   In a bowl, combine the chicken, sour cream, yogurt, mustard, and dill seasoning. Mix without breaking apart the chicken.

STEP 3   Cut the pita in half. Fill each side with ¼ cup of the lettuce, then add the chicken salad.

Makes 1 serving

Per serving: 192 calories, 26 g protein, 18 g carbohydrates, 2.5 g total fat, 0 g saturated fat, 3 g fiber, 410 mg sodium

TIP To give this dish extra nutritional punch, throw a small handful of raisins, dried cranberries, or unsalted sunflower seeds into the mix.

5-MINUTE CHICKEN SALAD SANDWICH

This is just as easy as the 2-Minute Chicken Salad Pita (page 73), and has celery, onion, and pine nuts added for crunch. It is full of muscle-building protein and clean enough to munch in any phase of your diet.

INGREDIENTS:

1   rib celery, finely chopped

1   tablespoon finely chopped onion

1   tablespoon pine nuts

1   heaping teaspoon spicy brown mustard

1   heaping teaspoon fat-free sour cream

1   heaping teaspoon fat-free plain yogurt
    Pinch of ground black pepper

2   cans (3 ounces each) chunk chicken, rinsed and drained twice

4   slices whole grain bread

2   leaves lettuce

HOW TO MAKE IT:

STEP 1 In a large bowl, mix together the celery, onion, pine nuts, mustard, sour cream, yogurt, and pepper.

STEP 2 Add the chicken and toss with the veggie mixture so you don't break it apart too much.

STEP 3 Spread half the chicken salad on a slice of bread. Add a lettuce leaf and top with another bread slice. Repeat with the remaining ingredients to make a second sandwich.

Makes 2 servings

Per serving: 267 calories, 28 g protein, 31 g carbohydrates, 5.5 g total fat, 0 g saturated fat, 11 g fiber, 410 mg sodium

DOUBLE-RINSING CANNED MEATS

According to the ESHA Nutrient Database, which follows stringent protocols for nutrient information, you can easily reduce the overall sodium content in canned meats like tuna, salmon, and chicken by as much as 30 percent just by draining the liquid from the can. I take it a step further—not just draining the liquid but always double-rinsing canned meats with water for good measure.

SIMPLE BAKED LEMON-PEPPER CHICKEN

This is one of those classic dinnertime meals. When I was growing up, if it was chicken night, this was the dish. You'll notice that in this recipe, I leave the skin on the chicken while it cooks. If you pull it off before baking, you'll lose the flavor and your chicken will come out as dry as particle board. So bake the chicken with the skin on and then pull it off before you chow down. The lemon-pepper flavor cooks down into the meat of the chicken.

INGREDIENTS:

4   chicken breasts with ribs and skin, rinsed and dried

2   teaspoons no-salt lemon-pepper seasoning

HOW TO MAKE IT:

STEP 1 Preheat the oven to 350°F.

STEP 2 Arrange the chicken rib side down in a 12" × 9" baking dish. Sprinkle with the lemon-pepper seasoning.

STEP 3 Bake for 1 hour, or until a thermometer inserted in the thickest portion registers 170°F and the juices run clear. Remove the skin and enjoy.

Makes 4 servings

Per serving: 130 calories, 27 g protein, 0 g carbohydrates, 1.5 g total fat, 0.5 g saturated fat, 0 g fiber, 77 mg sodium

SERVING SUGGESTION: Just like the Ripped Chicken (page 85), this recipe also yields zero carbs, which means you can serve it with a side of steamed veggies, wild rice, or a small amount of bow-tie pasta.

TIP I like to use a disposable aluminum baking pan with ridges to catch the grease and keep it away from the chicken as it cooks. You can also use a roasting pan and rack, but that means more cleanup.

ZESTY LEMON CHICKEN

INGREDIENTS:

6	lemons
4	boneless, skinless chicken breasts, rinsed, dried, and trimmed of fat
½	cup unbleached or all-purpose flour
1	teaspoon paprika
½	teaspoon ground black pepper
1	teaspoon extra-virgin olive oil
¼	cup water
1½	tablespoons brown sugar
	Pinch of no-salt lemon-pepper seasoning

HOW TO MAKE IT:

STEP 1 Halve the lemons and squeeze the juice of all but one half into a large bowl. Discard the juiced lemon rinds and set aside the ½ lemon.

STEP 2 Add the chicken to the lemon juice. Cover and refrigerate for 3 to 4 hours.

STEP 3 Preheat the oven to 350°F. In a shallow dish, mix together the flour, paprika, and pepper. Roll each chicken breast in the flour mix to lightly coat. (Discard the lemon juice.)

STEP 4 In a nonstick skillet, heat the oil to medium high and add the oil. Place the chicken in the skillet and brown for 2 minutes on each side. Remove the chicken to a 13" × 9" baking pan.

STEP 5 Add the water to the baking pan. Sprinkle the brown sugar over the chicken. Slice the reserved ½ lemon into 4 very thin slices. Lay one lemon slice over each chicken breast. Sprinkle with the lemon-pepper seasoning.

STEP 6 Bake for 45 minutes, or until a thermometer inserted in the thickest portion registers 160°F and the juices run clear.

Makes 4 servings

Per serving: 262 calories, 35 g protein, 24 g carbohydrates, 3 g total fat, 1 g saturated fat, 1 g fiber, 103 mg sodium

PINEAPPLE CHICKEN

INGREDIENTS:

1	teaspoon extra-virgin olive oil
¼	cup finely chopped sweet onion
	Pinch of ground black pepper
2	boneless, skinless chicken breasts, rinsed, dried, trimmed of fat, and cut into 1" cubes
1	tablespoon orange juice
1	can (8 ounces) pineapple chunks
1	banana, sliced
1	teaspoon maple syrup

HOW TO MAKE IT:

STEP 1 In a nonstick skillet over medium-high heat, add the oil, onion, and pepper. Cook for 1 minute, until the onion is slightly browned.

STEP 2 Stir in the chicken, orange juice, and pineapple (with juice).

STEP 3 Bring to a boil, then reduce the heat to medium.

STEP 4 Add the banana and syrup. Cook for 1 to 2 minutes.

STEP 5 Reduce the heat to low and stir. Cover and simmer for 5 minutes longer.

Makes 2 servings

Per serving: 288 calories, 28 g protein, 34 g carbohydrates, 4 g total fat, 1 g saturated fat, 3 g fiber, 88 mg sodium

SERVING SUGGESTION: Serve each breast over ½ cup brown or wild rice to help kick up the carbs, especially if you're chowing this meal post-workout.

GRILLED APRICOT-CHICKEN SKEWERS

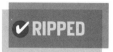

Ripe apricots have a wonderful sweet taste, and as a fruit preserve, their flavor is even more concentrated and enhanced. They're also high in potassium and carbs, so while the flavors are enticing, so too are the benefits as a postworkout snack. During a hard workout, you sweat out minerals like potassium and sodium, which results in muscle cramping and fatigue. After training, your muscles are primed for glycogen replenishment and need protein for tissue repair and growth. That's what makes this dish a helpful postworkout meal: The chicken offers a solid protein source, while the apricot preserves offer a boost of carbs to replenish glycogen stores and potassium to help restore lost minerals, helping prevent muscle cramping and fatigue.

INGREDIENTS:

½   cup 100% apricot whole-fruit preserves

2   tablespoons balsamic vinegar

2   tablespoons water

1   tablespoon toasted sesame oil

2   teaspoons dried sage

1   tablespoon honey (optional)

2   boneless, skinless chicken breasts, washed, trimmed of fat, and cut lengthwise into 8 long strips

        Pinch of ground black pepper

HOW TO MAKE IT:

STEP 1 Place 8 wooden skewers in a 13" × 9" baking pan and add water to cover.

STEP 2 In a large bowl, combine the preserves, vinegar, water, sesame oil, and sage and mix well. Pour half the marinade into a smaller bowl and reserve. This second bowl of marinade will be used to glaze the chicken while grilling. If it is not thick enough, add the honey and mix.

STEP 3 Add the chicken to the large bowl of marinade, cover, and refrigerate for 30 minutes.

STEP 4 Brush the grill rack with a little olive oil, or coat with cooking spray. Heat the grill to medium-low.

STEP 5 Insert a skewer through the length of each chicken strip. Discard the marinade.

STEP 6 Arrange the skewers on the grill. Sprinkle with the pepper. Cook for 20 minutes, turning twice and brushing several times with the smaller bowl of marinade to coat. Check for doneness by cutting into the center of one of the thickest pieces. The chicken should no longer be pink, and the juices should run clear.

Makes 4 servings

Per serving: 121 calories, 14 g protein, 11 g carbohydrates, 4 g total fat, 1 g saturated fat, 0 g fiber, 41 mg sodium

VARIATION: Cut the chicken into chunks, instead of strips, and skewer the chunks with pieces of red bell peppers and fresh pearl onions in between. Both the peppers and onions have a sweet taste that goes very well with the apricot glaze.

SERVING SUGGESTION: Serve with brown or wild rice, prepared according to the package directions, and grilled zucchini or yellow squash. Just cut the squash or zucchini in half, brush lightly with olive oil, sprinkle with a little pepper, and grill for 4 minutes per side. I always begin with the cut side down, then finish with the skin side down.

CHICKEN PICCATA

INGREDIENTS:

2	boneless, skinless ¼-inch-thick chicken cutlets, rinsed and dried
	Pinch of black pepper
½	cup unbleached or all-purpose flour
1	teaspoon extra-virgin olive oil
10	asparagus spears, with bottoms cut off
¼	cup dry white wine
2	tablespoons water
1	teaspoon minced garlic
	Juice of ½ lemon

HOW TO MAKE IT:

STEP 1 Sprinkle the chicken with pepper. In a shallow dish, roll each cutlet in the flour to coat.

STEP 2 In a nonstick skillet, heat the oil to medium-high. Add chicken. Cook the chicken for 1½ minutes per side, or until no longer pink and the juices run clear. Remove to a plate and set aside.

STEP 3 Reduce the heat to medium-low. In the skillet, combine the asparagus, wine, water, garlic, and lemon juice. Cook for 1½ to 2 minutes.

STEP 4 Return the chicken to the skillet. Cook for 1 minute on each side to coat with the sauce.

Makes 2 servings

Per serving: 350 calories, 36 g protein, 27 g carbohydrates, 4.5 g total fat, 1 g saturated fat, 1g fiber, 96 mg sodium

SERVING SUGGESTION: Lay each cutlet over ½ cup brown rice, then drizzle the sauce over top. I like to complement this dish with a simple salad like No-Prep Iceberg Wedges (page 172).

CHICKEN BREASTS VERSUS CUTLETS

What's the difference? The thickness. Boneless, skinless chicken breasts are much thicker than cutlets. That means they need more time to cook. Cutlets are sliced extra thin, so they cook quickly. If you buy cutlets that are still too thick, simply pound them to ¼-inch thickness.

CREAMY CHICKEN

INGREDIENTS:

2	boneless, skinless ¼-inch-thick chicken cutlets, rinsed and dried
	Pinch of ground black pepper
½	cup unbleached or all-purpose flour
1	teaspoon extra-virgin olive oil
1	small tomato, finely chopped
½	small yellow onion, chopped
¼	cup dry white wine
	Juice of ½ lemon
1	tablespoon half-and-half

HOW TO MAKE IT:

STEP 1 Sprinkle the chicken with the pepper. In a shallow dish, roll each cutlet in the flour to coat.

STEP 2 In a nonstick skillet, heat the oil to medium-high. Add the chicken. Cook the chicken for 1½ minutes per side, or until no longer pink and the juices run clear. Remove to a plate and set aside.

STEP 3 Reduce the heat to medium-low. In the skillet, combine the tomato, onion, wine, and lemon juice. Cook for 1 minute.

STEP 4 Reduce the heat to low. Add the half-and-half. Cook for 1 minute.

STEP 5 Return the chicken to the skillet. Cook for 1 minute on each side to coat with the sauce.

Makes 2 servings

Per serving: 364 calories, 37 g protein, 30 g carbohydrates, 5 g total fat, 1.5 g saturated fat, 1 g fiber, 101 mg sodium

SERVING SUGGESTION: Lay each cutlet over ½ cup brown rice, then drizzle the sauce over top. Eat with a side of Classic Steamed Veggies (page 154).

BAMBOO-STEAMED CHICKEN AND VEGGIES

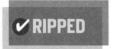

This dish requires a round, two-tier, 10" bamboo steamer, a piece of equipment you can find at any store that carries a wide range of cookware. (I picked mine up at the local mall.) The stackable tiers allow you to cook a few different foods at the same time. When I was preparing for bodybuilding contests, this was both the cooking tool and recipe that helped me get shredded. Be sure to get a pan that fits your 10" bamboo steamer. The steamer should fit snugly into the pan, with a little room around the edges to keep water and steam condensation from dripping onto the stove top and creating a mess. The best thing to do is to buy both the pan and the steamer together to ensure a proper fit.

INGREDIENTS:

4   boneless, skinless chicken breasts, rinsed, dried, and trimmed of fat

       No-salt lemon-pepper seasoning

2   zucchini, sliced into rounds

10   button mushrooms, sliced

2   cups broccoli florets

HOW TO MAKE IT:

STEP 1 Arrange the chicken in the lowest tier of the steamer. Sprinkle with the lemon-pepper seasoning (to taste). Cover with the steamer lid. Arrange the zucchini, mushrooms, and broccoli in the steamer's upper tier and set aside.

STEP 2 Pour 1" to 1½" of water into the pan that fits the steamer. Place the lowest steamer tier in the pan, making sure the water touches the bottom edge of the steamer to create a nice seal. Turn the heat to high and bring the water to a boil. Reduce the heat to medium high. Steam for 15 to 20 minutes.

STEP 3 Take the lid off the chicken, and add the upper steamer tier. Cover with the lid. Steam for 15 to 20 minutes, or until the vegetables are tender and a thermometer inserted in the thickest portion of the chicken registers 160°F and the juices run clear.

Makes 4 servings

Per serving: 191 calories, 36 g protein, 7 g carbohydrates, 2 g total fat, .5 g saturated fat, 2.5 g fiber, 121 mg sodium

For easier cleanup and to keep the chicken from sticking to the bamboo steamer, you can place a lettuce leaf under the chicken.

ROSEMARY CHICKEN WITH VEGETABLES

INGREDIENTS:

1	teaspoon extra-virgin olive oil
2	potatoes, peeled and cut into cubes
1	can (14 ounces) no-salt chicken broth
4	boneless, skinless chicken breasts, rinsed, dried, and trimmed of fat
10–12	grape or cherry tomatoes
1	handful fresh green beans, trimmed of stems
1	yellow onion, finely chopped
1	rib celery, finely chopped
¼	cup dry white wine
	Juice of ½ lemon
½	teaspoon dried sage
½	teaspoon dried rosemary
½	teaspoon dried or fresh parsley
¼	teaspoon ground black pepper

HOW TO MAKE IT:

STEP 1 Preheat the oven to 450°F. In a 13" × 9" baking dish, combine the oil and potatoes. Toss to lightly coat the potatoes with oil. Bake for 15 minutes, or until the potatoes are slightly browned.

STEP 2 Add the broth, chicken, tomatoes, beans, onion, celery, wine, and lemon juice. Sprinkle with the sage, rosemary, parsley, and pepper.

STEP 3 Cover with foil and bake for 40 minutes.

STEP 4 Uncover and bake for 10 to 15 minutes longer, or until a thermometer inserted in the thickest portion of the chicken registers 160°F and the juices run clear.

Makes 4 servings

Per serving: 287 calories, 37 g protein, 22 g carbohydrates, 4 g total fat, 1 g saturated fat, 3 g fiber, 167 mg sodium

BURMESE CHICKEN CURRY

This is one of my favorite dishes to bring people together. It fills the house with an aroma so savory you'll have the neighbors calling. You'll soon have a free-for-all of delectable food, conversation, and good times! With muscle-building protein, and relatively low fat and sodium content, this recipe is good enough for all your health-conscious friends and family. The curry and turmeric spices are loaded with antioxidant and blood-cleansing properties, including anti-inflammatory and anti-aging compounds.

INGREDIENTS:

3–5	teaspoons cornstarch
3–5	teaspoons water
4	pounds boneless, skinless chicken breasts, rinsed, dried, trimmed of fat, and cut into 1" cubes
2½	cups water
3	tablespoons extra-virgin olive oil
7	ribs celery, chopped
2	apples, chopped
2	cloves garlic, minced
½	cup finely chopped sweet onions
2	tablespoons low-sodium soy sauce
4	teaspoons curry powder
2	teaspoons turmeric
2	teaspoons powdered ginger
1 or 2	dashes ground red pepper

HOW TO MAKE IT:

STEP 1 In a small dish, mix 1 teaspoon of the cornstarch with 1 tablespoon of the water until the cornstarch has completely dissolved. Repeat with the remaining cornstarch and water. Set aside.

STEP 2 In a large pot over medium-high heat, combine the rest of the ingredients. Add 1 teaspoon of the reserved cornstarch slurry and stir thoroughly. Bring to a quiet boil.

STEP 3 Reduce the heat to low and cover. Cook for 40 minutes to 1 hour, stirring every 15 minutes to check for consistency, adding another teaspoon or two of the cornstarch slurry to help thicken the liquid. Add a little more curry powder to taste as the recipe simmers.

Makes 8 servings

Per serving: 352 calories, 54 g protein, 14 g carbohydrates, 8 g total fat, 1.5 g saturated fat, 3 g fiber, 329 mg sodium

HOW TO SERVE: Ladle each serving of curry over ½ cup white rice. Serve with the following as condiments: finely chopped onions, chopped hard-cooked eggs, raisins, crushed unsalted roasted almonds, chopped bananas, chopped apples, and hot and sweet chutneys.

RIPPED CHICKEN

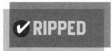
✔ RIPPED

INGREDIENTS:

2   boneless, skinless chicken breasts, rinsed, dried, and trimmed of fat

1   teaspoon McCormick Salt Free All-Purpose Seasoning

HOW TO MAKE IT:

STEP 1 Preheat the oven to 350°F.

STEP 2 Arrange the chicken breasts in a baking dish. Sprinkle with the seasoning.

STEP 3 Bake for 30 minutes, or until a thermometer inserted in the thickest portion registers 160°F and the juices run clear.

Makes 2 servings

Per serving: 156 calories, 33 g protein, 0 g carbohydrates, 2 g total fat, 0.5 g saturated fat, 0 g fiber, 92 mg sodium

VARIATIONS: Instead of all-purpose seasoning, you can substitute one of the following: 1 teaspoon no-salt lemon-pepper seasoning; ¼ teaspoon each dried basil, dried thyme, dried rosemary, and ground black pepper; ¼ cup no-salt pasta sauce and ¼ cup water; or ½ cup no-salt chicken broth and a dash of pepper.

TIP For easy grab-and-go meals, double or triple the recipe; wait until the chicken breasts have cooled, then throw each into a separate zip-top bag and store in the fridge for up to 4 days.

FRIED CHICKEN, MUSCLE-CHOW STYLE

Conventional fried chicken starts with healthy lean protein—but then

it's rolled in a crust of empty carbs and set afloat in a vat of boiling

saturated fat. Not my idea of finger-lickin' good! I designed the

following three recipes as a healthy alternative. They call for a simple

breading technique that allows you to achieve a crispy coating without

frying. It's just as flavorful, and you'll see that you can enjoy crispy

chicken without all the unnecessary oil and added fat.

HIGH-PROTEIN PAN-COOKED CHICKEN

INGREDIENTS:

2	eggs, beaten
1	tablespoon fat-free milk
1	cup 4C Carb Careful Plain Breadcrumbs
1	tablespoon grated Parmesan cheese
1	teaspoon dried basil
4	boneless, skinless ¼-inch-thick chicken cutlets, rinsed and dried
1	teaspoon extra-virgin olive oil

HOW TO MAKE IT:

STEP 1 In a shallow dish, mix together the eggs and milk.

STEP 2 In another shallow dish, mix together the bread crumbs, cheese, and basil.

STEP 3 Dredge each cutlet in the egg mixture, then roll in the bread crumb mixture to coat.

STEP 4 In a nonstick skillet, heat the oil to medium high. Cook the chicken for 4 minutes per side, or until no longer pink and the juices run clear.

Makes 2 servings

Per serving: 533 calories, 88 g protein, 15 g carbohydrates, 11 g total fat, 3 g saturated fat, 8 g fiber, 273 mg sodium

CRISPY CHICKEN

This recipe gets its crunch from cornflakes. Since I don't eat much cereal, I buy the single-serving boxes rather than have a large open box sitting in the cabinet going stale.

INGREDIENTS:

2	tablespoons spicy brown mustard
3	teaspoons apple cider vinegar
1	teaspoon hot-pepper sauce
1	teaspoon brown sugar
1	can (5 ounces) evaporated milk
2	single-serving boxes cornflakes, pulverized into small pieces
½	cup 4C Carb Careful Plain Breadcrumbs
½	teaspoon paprika
4	boneless, skinless chicken breasts, rinsed, dried, and pounded to an even thickness (see note)
1	teaspoon extra-virgin olive oil

HOW TO MAKE IT:

STEP 1 Preheat the oven to 350°F. In a shallow dish, mix together the mustard, vinegar, hot-pepper sauce, and brown sugar. Add the evaporated milk and stir with a fork for about 30 seconds, or until thick.

STEP 2 In another shallow dish, mix together the cornflakes, bread crumbs, and paprika.

STEP 3 Dredge each chicken breast in the milk mixture, then roll in the cornflake mixture to coat.

STEP 4 Coat a 12" × 9" baking dish with the oil. Add the chicken. Bake for 1 hour, or until a thermometer inserted in the thickest portion registers 160°F and the juices run clear.

Makes 4 servings

Per serving: 325 calories, 43 g protein, 24 g carbohydrates, 6 g total fat, 2.5 g saturated fat, 3 g fiber, 359 mg sodium

SERVING SUGGESTION: No-Prep Iceberg Wedges (page 172) goes nicely with this dish.

NOTE To ensure even cooking when preparing boneless chicken breasts, place each breast between two pieces of plastic wrap and gently pound with the flat side of a meat tenderizer or mallet until they are of even thickness. If you don't own a meat tenderizer or mallet, you can just as easily use the bottom of a small pot or the bottom of a wine bottle.

SPICY CHICKEN CUTLETS

INGREDIENTS:

2	eggs, beaten
1	tablespoon fat-free milk
1	cup 4C Carb Careful Plain Breadcrumbs
1	teaspoon dried minced onion
1	teaspoon dried oregano
½	teaspoon ground red pepper
¼	teaspoon paprika
¼	teaspoon ground black pepper
4	boneless, skinless ¼-inch-thick chicken cutlets, rinsed and dried
1	teaspoon extra-virgin olive oil

HOW TO MAKE IT:

STEP 1 In a shallow dish, mix together the eggs and milk.

STEP 2 In another shallow dish, mix together the bread crumbs, onion, oregano, red pepper, paprika, and black pepper.

STEP 3 Dredge each cutlet in the egg mixture, then roll in the bread crumb mixture to coat.

STEP 4 In a nonstick skillet, heat the oil to medium high. Add the chicken. Cook the chicken for 4 minutes on each side, or until a thermometer inserted in the thickest portion registers 160°F and the juices run clear.

Makes 4 servings

Per serving: 322 calories, 55 g protein, 8 g carbohydrates, 6 g total fat, 1.5 g saturated fat, 4 g fiber, 151 mg sodium

SERVING SUGGESTION: Slice the chicken and serve on a bed of prewashed mixed greens. Top with Creamy Honey-Mustard Dressing (page 181).

6

TURKEY

Turkey isn't just for Thanksgiving. It can be used to replace ground beef in meat loaf, spaghetti sauce, chili, hamburgers, and meatballs. And it's one of the most popular deli meats out there. As is true of chicken, this white meat is chock-full of muscle-building protein that's low in fat and contains zero carbs.

I've compiled some of my favorite ways to prepare this versatile bird, so if you're trying to cut your red meat consumption, this chapter gives you some great options.

MUSCLE-T BURGERS

INGREDIENTS:

¼   cup 4C® Carb Careful Plain
       Breadcrumbs

10   fresh basil leaves, chopped

2   tablespoons chopped yellow onion

2   tablespoons chopped dried or
       fresh parsley

2   tablespoons grated Parmesan cheese

1   pound extra-lean ground turkey breast

1   egg white
       Pinch of garlic powder
       Coarse ground black pepper

4   whole grain burger buns (buy the
       lowest-sodium buns you can find)

1   bag (4 ounces) prewashed arugula

1   large tomato, thinly sliced

¼   cup low-sodium pasta sauce

HOW TO MAKE IT:

STEP 1 In a large bowl, combine the bread crumbs, basil, onion, parsley, and cheese. Mix with a fork.

STEP 2 Add the turkey and egg white. Use your hands to mix well.

STEP 3 Form into four ½"-thick patties. Sprinkle with the garlic powder and pepper (to taste).

STEP 4 Grill over medium heat for 15 to 18 minutes, turning once halfway through, or until a thermometer inserted in the center registers 165°F and the meat is no longer pink.

STEP 5 While the burgers are cooking, add the buns to the grill until lightly toasted. In a small microwaveable bowl, microwave the pasta sauce for 1 minute.

STEP 6 Slide each burger onto a bun. Top with some arugula, a tomato slice, and 1 tablespoon of the pasta sauce.

Makes 4 servings

Per serving: 353 calories, 52 g protein, 25 g carbohydrates, 5 g total fat, 1 g saturated fat, 4 g fiber, 505 mg sodium

VEGGIE-TURKEY MEAT LOAF

INGREDIENTS:

1	pound extra-lean ground turkey breast
2	egg whites
1	medium zucchini, coarsely grated
1	bunch fresh parsley, chopped (about ⅓ cup)
1	can (8.5 ounces) no-salt sweet peas, rinsed and drained
½	sweet onion, chopped
½	cup shredded carrots
½	cup 4C Carb Careful Plain Breadcrumbs
½	teaspoon McCormick Salt Free All-Purpose Seasoning
½	cup low-sodium pasta sauce

HOW TO MAKE IT:

STEP 1 Preheat the oven to 350°F. In a large bowl, combine all the ingredients except ¼ cup of the pasta sauce. Use your hands to mix together well.

STEP 2 Coat a nonstick 9" × 5" loaf pan with cooking spray. Wipe away any excess spray with a paper towel.

STEP 3 Place the meat mixture in the pan and shape from edge to edge so it's even. Bake for 45 minutes.

STEP 4 Pour the remaining ¼ cup pasta sauce over the top, spreading evenly with the back of a spoon. Bake for 16 minutes longer, or until a thermometer inserted in the center registers 165°F and the meat is no longer pink.

STEP 5 Cool for 10 minutes before slicing.

Makes 7 servings

Per serving: 128 calories, 22 g protein, 8 g carbohydrates, 1 g total fat, 0 g saturated fat, 3 g fiber, 80 mg sodium

SERVING SUGGESTION: For the classic feel of a home-cooked meat loaf dinner, prepare a side of plain instant mashed potatoes. I always buy 100 percent real Idaho potatoes with no fat and very low sodium. I prepare them on the stove according to the package directions, with a little McCormick Imitation Butter Flavor or a fat-free butter spray mixed in. They are easy to make and take only minutes.

TIP The best part of making meat loaf is that the leftovers make a great on-the-go meal anytime, warm or cold. Meat loaf will keep in the fridge for three days without a problem. Throw a slice between two pieces of whole grain bread and top with a spoonful of low-sodium pasta sauce for a great postworkout meal.

OVEN-BAKED TURKEY MEATBALLS

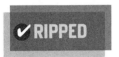

These meatballs make a great high-protein on-the-go snack that you can throw into a baggie and take on the road. You can also make them into a meal—easily. Just throw 4 meatballs and 1 cup of no-salt tomato sauce (per person) into a saucepan and warm over medium heat. Serve them over ½ cup of pasta.

INGREDIENTS:

1½	**pounds extra-lean ground turkey breast**
2	**egg whites**
½	**cup toasted wheat germ**
¼	**cup quick-cooking oats**
1	**tablespoon whole flaxseeds**
1	**tablespoon grated Parmesan cheese**
½	**teaspoon McCormick Salt Free All-Purpose Seasoning**
¼	**teaspoon ground black pepper**

HOW TO MAKE IT:

STEP 1 Preheat the oven to 400°F. Coat a 2-quart baking dish with cooking spray.

STEP 2 Place all the ingredients in a large bowl and mix together well with your hands. Shape the mixture into 16 to 20 golf ball–sized meatballs and place them in the baking dish.

STEP 3 Bake for 7 minutes. Turn the meatballs, then bake for 8 to 13 minutes longer, or until no longer pink.

Makes 4 servings

Per serving (4 meatballs): 282 calories, 50 g protein, 12 g carbohydrates, 6 g total fat, 0.5 g saturated fat, 3.5 g fiber, 146 mg sodium

TIP For uniformly sized meatballs, use an ice cream scoop to form each one. This will also ensure they cook evenly.

RIPPED TIP

If you make these meatballs during a Ripped Phase, it's best to separate them into zip-top bags (4 meatballs in each) to control your portions. Then store the extras in the fridge so you have several high-protein grab-and-go meals throughout the week.

TURKEY AND BROCCOLI WITH COUSCOUS

Have all your ingredients ready because this meal cooks very fast—15 minutes from beginning to end.

INGREDIENTS:

¼   **red bell pepper, cut into thin strips**

1–2   **tablespoons chopped yellow onion**

       Pinch of ground black pepper

½   **pound boneless, skinless turkey cutlets, rinsed, dried, and sliced into 2" strips**

1   **teaspoon dried sage**

1   **cup low-sodium, fat-free chicken broth**

1   **cup broccoli florets**

½   **cup couscous**

HOW TO MAKE IT:

STEP 1 Coat a deep skillet with cooking spray. Wipe away any excess spray with a paper towel. Heat the skillet over medium heat.

STEP 2 Add the bell pepper, onion, and black pepper and cook, stirring frequently, for 2 minutes, or until the onion is slightly translucent.

STEP 3 Add the turkey and sage. Cook for 2 minutes.

STEP 4 Add the broth and broccoli. Bring to a boil for 1 minute.

STEP 5 Stir in the couscous.

STEP 6 Cover the skillet and remove from the heat for 5 to 10 minutes, or until the couscous has absorbed all of the broth. Stir and serve.

Makes 4 servings

Per serving: 157 calories, 18 g protein, 19 g carbohydrates, 1 g total fat, 0 g saturated fat, 2 g fiber, 92 mg sodium

NO-BRAINER ROASTED TURKEY

For some guys, roasting a turkey can be an intimidating task—but not anymore. Whether you're entertaining some friends, spending the holiday season solo, or just looking to bake a bird anytime of the year, this is one of the easiest meals you'll ever make. The best part is that you can have fresh-carved, high-protein turkey all week long to throw on a salad, in a sandwich, or into a baggie and then your gym bag.

INGREDIENTS:

3   **pounds frozen boneless, skinless turkey breast**

1   **teaspoon extra-virgin olive oil**

½   **teaspoon no-salt lemon-pepper seasoning**

HOW TO MAKE IT:

STEP 1   Preheat the oven to 350°F. Brush the bottom of the turkey with ½ teaspoon of the oil and place it in a roasting pan. Brush the rest of the turkey with the remaining ½ teaspoon oil. Sprinkle with the lemon-pepper seasoning.

STEP 2   Roast for 2 hours (or for the time specified on the package directions), or until a thermometer inserted in the thickest portion registers 170°F and the juices run clear.

STEP 3   Remove from the oven and set aside for 15 minutes. To carve, cut off the netting, remove the skin, and slice.

Makes 12 servings

Per serving (3.5 ounces): 85 calories, 19 g protein, 0 g carbohydrates, 1 g total fat, 0 g saturated fat, 0 g fiber, 370 mg sodium

TIP   A Butterball turkey breast will come with a gravy packet that I toss in the garbage. Keep in mind that the nutritional information on the Butterball package includes this gravy packet—eliminate it and you improve the overall nutritional profile by a landslide. Store leftover turkey in the fridge for use throughout the week.

PREWORKOUT TURKEY SANDWICH

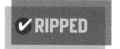

I've heard people say that training on an empty stomach, first thing in the morning, helps burn more fat. It's true that a workout like this can blow through your glycogen stores in less than an hour, and after that time your body will look to fat stores for usable energy. But there are two problems that I've experienced with this strategy: a lack of energy, and the fact that your body will also start to burn muscle tissue as an energy source. So how can you burn fat and not lose muscle in the process? The answer is simple: Eat a well-designed preworkout meal that allows you to walk that tightrope during your training sessions. An ideal preworkout meal should:

1. Contain an easily digestible protein. The protein will fuel your muscles during training.

2. Be low in fat. Fat slows digestion and interferes with vasodilation. That means less blood pumping nutrients into your muscles, higher lactic acid levels in the muscle, and slower recovery between sets, as well as difficulty achieving a pump.

3. Be moderate to low in fiber, but not highly glycemic either. A high-glycemic meal can spike insulin levels and cause a mood crash prior to your workout. Too much fiber can make you feel full, bloated, and heavy. Just enough will give you sustained energy to last throughout a grueling workout.

This sandwich will fuel your body before you even walk into the gym. And it will set the stage for optimum fat burning, while helping avoid muscle catabolism. Eat it 1 hour before your workout.

INGREDIENTS:

1   teaspoon honey mustard (use the lowest-sodium one you can find)

2   slices Ezekiel 4:9 Organic Sprouted 100% Whole Grain Flourless Low Sodium Bread

2   ounces low-sodium turkey breast, thinly sliced

2   thin slices tomato

1   small handful alfalfa sprouts or shredded lettuce

HOW TO MAKE IT:

STEP 1 Spread the mustard onto the bread slices.

STEP 2 On one of the slices, stack the turkey, tomato, and sprouts or lettuce.

STEP 3 Top with the second bread slice.

Makes 1 serving

Per serving: 279 calories, 27 g protein, 38 g carbohydrates, 2 g total fat, 0 g saturated fat, 8 g fiber, 101 mg sodium

7

EGGS

Good things come in small packages, and eggs are an integral part of the Muscle Chow diet. They are relatively inexpensive and can be eaten anytime of the day. Known as a popular breakfast food, they also wind up on salads for lunch, as egg salad at barbecues, deviled for snacks, and served for dinner at 24-hour diners across the country. Eggs are loaded with quality protein for building muscle; omega-3 fatty acids for healthy joints and skin, inflammation reduction, and overall health; zinc and cholesterol for hormone (i.e., testosterone) production; lecithin for fat metabolism and improved vascularity; and choline to support brain function. They've also got antioxidant vitamins like

SODIUM IN EGGS

You'll notice slightly higher amounts of sodium in the following egg recipes than in most of the other recipes in this book. Don't be alarmed—this is due to the naturally occurring sodium in eggs. Your body more readily assimilates this sodium than it does the common iodized table salt that has been refined and stripped of any nutritional value.

A, B, D, and E, plus the mineral selenium—all of which fight free radicals and increase energy production.

Glycemically speaking, eggs are a nonfactor. This means you can add carbs to most egg recipes and maintain a favorable nutritional balance that won't spike insulin levels.

Here's the key though: While many people are afraid of eating the yolks because of their fat and cholesterol content, that's exactly where most of the other crucial nutrients are found. For instance, the yolk contains almost half of an egg's protein, with 2.75 grams. Fortunately, studies show that the cholesterol in eggs has little to no effect on your body's serum cholesterol levels.

That said, I'm not recommending that you eat a dozen whole eggs every morning. On the Muscle Chow diet, you want to control the amount of fat you consume in order to maintain a lean physique and six-pack abs. That's why—as a rule—you'll find that most of the egg recipes in this book call for just one or two egg yolks for every six eggs. However, you can increase or reduce this ratio depending on what phase of a diet cycle you're in. In a Relaxed Phase or Lean Phase, having one or two egg yolks along with the whites is fine. On the other hand, in a more strict Ripped Phase portion of a diet cycle, you might decide to stick with just one egg yolk or go with all whites to eliminate the fat altogether. Adjust the recipes as you need to. For example, if a recipe calls for one whole egg and five egg whites (like the Giant Omelet Scramble on page 101), you can easily increase or reduce the number of yolks by one. And to increase the protein content of a dish by 4 grams, you can always add an extra egg white.

One final note before we get cracking: I use large omega-3-fortified eggs in all my recipes.

SEPARATE WAYS

I've found that the best way to separate an egg yolk from the white is to simply use your hands. Sure, there are specific tools for the job, but using them means more cleanup and more gadgets cluttering up your utensil drawer. Here's how I do it: Crack the eggs into a bowl, being careful not to break the yolks. Using your fingers, scoop out one yolk at a time and very gently roll it across your fingers in both hands, allowing the whites to fall through and back into the bowl.

CLEAN FRIED EGGS

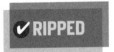

This is one of my favorite evening snacks, offering a solid amount of muscle-building protein plus a healthy portion of saturated fat and cholesterol to help boost testosterone levels. Maybe it's all in my head, but when I chow this dish before bed, I swear I can feel a difference the next morning—in both energy and muscle size. The whole grain bread in this recipe causes less of an insulin response than refined bread, helping to slow digestion. If you want to slow down the absorption rate a little more, top off each slice of toast with a little flaxseed oil (see "A Toast to Muscle Growth" on page 100).

INGREDIENTS:

2	eggs
4	egg whites
	Dash of ground black pepper
2	slices Ezekiel 4:9 Organic Sprouted 100% Whole Grain Flourless Low Sodium Bread, toasted

HOW TO MAKE IT:

STEP 1 Coat a nonstick skillet with cooking spray, then lightly wipe away the excess spray with a paper towel. Heat the skillet over medium heat.

STEP 2 Add the eggs and egg whites and top with the black pepper. Cover and cook for 3 to 4 minutes, or until the yolks turn pink and the whites are just firm.

STEP 3 Slide the eggs onto a plate, along with the toast.

Makes 1 serving

Per serving: 398 calories, 36 g protein, 36 g carbohydrates, 11 g total fat, 3 g saturated fat, 7 g fiber, 362 mg sodium

RIPPED TIP
Have this dish no more than twice a week when you're in a Ripped Phase.

TIP Use a skillet with a glass lid so you can see the doneness of the eggs without lifting the lid and releasing the steam.

DIRTY EGGS

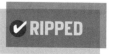 **RIPPED**

These aren't pretty, but they serve a purpose—they supply solid protein and fiber, the two things I look for when I'm eating to get ripped. It's what I call "food with a function."

INGREDIENTS:

1	egg
5	egg whites
¼	cup unprocessed wheat bran
	Pinch of ground black pepper

HOW TO MAKE IT:

STEP 1 In a bowl, whisk the egg and egg whites until frothy. Add the bran and let it soak for 3 to 5 minutes.

STEP 2 Coat a skillet with cooking spray, then lightly wipe away the excess spray with a paper towel. Heat the skillet over medium-high heat.

STEP 3 Pour the egg mixture into the skillet and stir until the eggs begin to set. Once they start to set, cook for about 30 seconds without stirring, then stir to scramble for 3 to 4 minutes, or until fully cooked.

Makes 1 serving

Per serving: 191 calories, 27 g protein, 12 g carbohydrates, 5 g total fat, 1.5 g saturated fat, 6 g fiber, 347 mg sodium

A TOAST TO MUSCLE GROWTH

Besides being a traditional part of breakfast, toast is one of my favorite snacks anytime of the day. Toast a slice or two of whole grain bread, then drizzle a teaspoon of flaxseed oil over each slice. Using a butter knife, press down on the toast to help the oil soak in, then cut each slice in half. The crunchy texture of the crust blended with the nutty flaxseed flavor makes this healthy, omega-3-rich, whole grain snack addictive. To help balance out the glycemic impact of this snack, add a protein source. I'll often have a 90% Shake (page 190) or a pop-top can of chicken (double-rinsed).

GIANT OMELET SCRAMBLE

INGREDIENTS:

1	egg
5	egg whites
3	tablespoons instant potato flakes
3	tablespoons water
1	tablespoon finely chopped onion
	Pinch of ground black pepper
½	small tomato, seeded, chopped, and drained of excess juice
1	heaping tablespoon low-fat feta cheese crumbles

HOW TO MAKE IT:

STEP 1 In a bowl, whisk together the egg, egg whites, potato flakes, and water.

STEP 2 Coat a skillet with cooking spray and heat over medium heat. Add the onion and pepper. Cook for 1 minute. Reduce the heat to medium-low.

STEP 3 Add the tomato to the egg mixture. Pour into the skillet. Lightly stir until the egg mixture begins to set.

STEP 4 Cook without stirring for 2 minutes, or until the eggs start to look firm. Using a spatula, flip the omelet.

STEP 5 Add the cheese and fold the omelet in half. Cook for 30 seconds. Flip and cook for 30 seconds longer.

Makes 1 serving

Per serving: 223 calories, 28 g protein, 12 g carbohydrates, 6.5 g total fat, 2 g saturated fat, 2 g fiber, 480 mg sodium

SERVING SUGGESTION: Pair the omelet with a slice of whole grain toast lightly coated with a little fat-free pump-spray butter. If you're looking to increase stamina or replenish glycogen stores, the toast will help boost the carbs slightly.

SPANISH EGG SCRAMBLE

INGREDIENTS:

½	potato, peeled
1	egg
5	egg whites
1	tablespoon chopped red bell pepper
1	tablespoon chopped green bell pepper
1	tablespoon chopped onion
	Pinch of black pepper
	Dash of hot-pepper sauce

HOW TO MAKE IT:

STEP 1 Wrap the potato in a paper towel and microwave on high for 4 minutes, or until you can easily insert a fork through to the middle. Set aside. When the potato is cool, grate it.

STEP 2 In a bowl, whisk together the egg and egg whites until frothy.

STEP 3 Coat a skillet with cooking spray and heat over medium-high heat. Add the grated potato, red and green bell peppers, onion, black pepper, and hot-pepper sauce. Cook for 3 to 4 minutes.

STEP 4 Reduce the heat to medium. Add the egg mixture. Cook, stirring to scramble, for 3 to 4 minutes, or until the eggs are firm.

Makes 1 serving

Per serving: 228 calories, 26 g protein, 17 g carbohydrates, 5.5 g total fat, 1.5 g saturated fat, 2 g fiber, 353 mg sodium

SERVING SUGGESTION: Pair the scrambled eggs with a slice of whole grain toast lightly coated with a little fat-free pump-spray butter. If you're looking to increase stamina or replenish glycogen stores, the toast will help boost the carbs slightly.

EASY WESTERN OMELET

INGREDIENTS:

1	**egg**
5	**egg whites**
3	**tablespoons water or fat-free milk**
1	**tablespoon finely chopped onion**
1	**tablespoon finely chopped red bell pepper**
4	**white mushrooms, sliced**
	Pinch of ground black pepper
1	**teaspoon grated Parmesan cheese**

HOW TO MAKE IT:

STEP 1 In a bowl, whisk together the egg, egg whites, and water or milk.

STEP 2 Coat a skillet with cooking spray and heat over medium heat. Add the onion, bell pepper, mushrooms, and black pepper. Cook for 1 minute. Reduce the heat to medium-low.

STEP 3 Add the egg mixture. Cook, stirring, until the egg mixture begins to set. Cook without stirring for 2 minutes, or until the eggs start to look firm. Flip the omelet.

STEP 4 Add the cheese and fold the omelet in half. Cook for 30 seconds. Flip and cook for 30 seconds longer.

Makes 1 serving

Per serving: 190 calories, 28 g protein, 6 g carbohydrates, 6 g total fat, 2 g saturated fat, 1 g fiber, 378 mg sodium

SERVING SUGGESTION: Because this recipe is low in carbs, you might choose to add pan-cooked hash browns as a side dish. Be sure to get the lowest-sodium, lowest-fat potatoes you can find (refrigerated or frozen). Brown in a skillet with a little parsley and ground black pepper.

EGG WHITE MORNING WRAP

INGREDIENTS:

6	egg whites
¼	cup water or fat-free milk
	Pinch of ground black pepper
	Pinch of dried or fresh basil
1	whole wheat tortilla (choose the lowest fat and sodium brand you can find)

HOW TO MAKE IT:

STEP 1 In a bowl, whisk together the egg whites, water or milk, pepper, and basil.

STEP 2 Coat a skillet with cooking spray, then lightly wipe away the excess spray with a paper towel. Heat the skillet over medium heat.

STEP 3 Add the egg mixture. Cook, stirring, for 3 to 4 minutes, or until firm.

STEP 4 Microwave the tortilla for 30 seconds.

STEP 5 Place the eggs on the tortilla and roll up burrito style.

Makes 1 serving

Per serving: 185 calories, 27 g protein, 13 g carbohydrates, 2.5 g total fat, 0 g saturated fat, 2 g fiber, 514 mg sodium

SERVING SUGGESTION: Top with some Metabolic Salsa (see page 223).

VARIATION: For a smaller wrap, use four egg whites instead of six and only 2 tablespoons of water or milk.

MORNING PITA

INGREDIENTS:

4	white mushrooms, sliced
1	tablespoon chopped onion
1	tablespoon chopped red bell pepper
	Pinch of ground black pepper
1	egg
3	egg whites
½	small tomato, seeded and chopped
3	tablespoons water or fat-free milk
1	whole wheat pita (choose the lowest fat and sodium brand you can find), halved and toasted
½	avocado, sliced

HOW TO MAKE IT:

STEP 1 Coat a skillet with cooking spray. Heat over medium heat. Add the mushrooms, onion, bell pepper, and black pepper. Cook for 3 to 4 minutes.

STEP 2 Meanwhile, in a bowl, combine the egg, egg whites, tomato, and water or milk. Whisk together until frothy.

STEP 3 Pour the egg mixture into the skillet. Cook, stirring, for 3 to 4 minutes, or until the eggs are firm.

STEP 4 Fill each pita pocket with half the eggs.

Makes 1 serving

Per serving: 401 calories, 25 g protein, 33 g carbohydrates, 21 g total fat, 4 g saturated fat, 11 g fiber, 416 mg sodium

SERVING SUGGESTION: Serve with a side of sliced avocado.

MATZO BREI

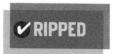 **✔ RIPPED**

This is one of my all-time favorite dishes. The matzos add just the right flavor and texture to make this a satiating treat anytime. Give it a try and see for yourself. Look for matzo in the kosher section of your grocery store.

INGREDIENTS:

1	egg
5	egg whites
2	or 3 sheets unsalted matzos
	Pinch of sea salt (optional)

HOW TO MAKE IT:

STEP 1 In a bowl, whisk together the egg and egg whites.

STEP 2 Run each matzo under warm tap water for 30 seconds, or until soggy. Crumble them into the eggs and mix well.

STEP 3 Coat a skillet with cooking spray, then wipe away the excess spray with a paper towel. Heat the skillet over medium-high heat.

STEP 4 Add the matzo-egg mixture. Cook, stirring, for 3 to 4 minutes, or until the eggs are firm. Add the sea salt (if using).

Makes 1 serving

Per serving: 380 calories, 30 g protein, 50 g carbohydrates, 5 g total fat, 2 g saturated fat, 0 g fiber, 347 mg sodium

RIPPED TIP

To lower the carb content, only use two sheets of matzo when in a Ripped Phase.

SPICY EGGS 'N' OATS SCRAMBLE

INGREDIENTS:

1	egg
4	egg whites
½	cup oats
¼	teaspoon dried basil or 1 tablespoon fresh
	Pinch of ground black pepper
⅓	cup chopped tomatoes
⅓	cup chopped fresh baby spinach (about 10 leaves)
1	teaspoon finely chopped onion
1	teaspoon grated Parmesan cheese
	Dash of hot-pepper sauce

HOW TO MAKE IT:

STEP 1 In a bowl, whisk together the egg and egg whites until frothy.

STEP 2 Add the oats, basil, and pepper. Allow to soak for 3 minutes.

STEP 3 Coat a skillet with cooking spray, then wipe away the excess spray with a paper towel. Heat the skillet over medium heat.

STEP 4 Add the egg mixture and cook for 30 seconds.

STEP 5 Add the tomatoes, spinach, and onion. Cook, stirring, for 3 to 4 minutes, or until the eggs are firm.

STEP 6 Remove to a plate and top with the cheese and hot-pepper sauce.

Makes 1 serving

Per serving: 334 calories, 28 g protein, 34 g carbohydrates, 9 g total fat, 2 g saturated fat, 5 g fiber, 340 mg sodium

RISE 'N' SHINE, IT'S TIME TO GET ANABOLIC

Breakfast is the first of two important opportunities in your day to chow some quick-digesting high-GI carbs (the next is postworkout). After you wake from an 8-hour slumber without a morsel of nutrition, chances are your body will be close to a catabolic state. Your glycogen stores are close to empty, and your body will begin using muscle as energy if you don't break the cycle. This is the perfect time to douse your system with a high-GI food to trigger an insulin response and halt that process. So if you're chowing a half dozen eggs at your first meal of the day, it's a good idea to also have two slices of wheat toast topped off with some whole fruit preserves. This will give your body and your muscles exactly what they need to get you back into an anabolic state at the onset of your day.

EGG SALAD SANDWICH

INGREDIENTS:

2	hard-cooked eggs (see Hard-Cooked Eggs by the Dozen on page 109)
4	hard-cooked egg whites
2	tablespoons fat-free sour cream
2	tablespoons finely chopped onion
1	heaping tablespoon Bookbinder's Chipotle Mustard (see note)
¼	teaspoon dried dill
	Dash of ground black pepper
4	slices whole grain bread, toasted

HOW TO MAKE IT:

STEP 1 In a bowl, use a potato masher to mash the eggs and egg whites into small pieces.

STEP 2 Add the sour cream, onion, mustard, dill, and pepper. Stir until well mixed.

STEP 3 Spread half the egg salad on 2 slices of the toast. Complete each sandwich with another slice of toast.

Makes 2 servings

Per serving: 226 calories, 19 g protein, 23 g carbohydrates, 6 g total fat, 1.5 g saturated fat, 4 g fiber, 193 mg sodium

TIP Bookbinder's Chipotle Mustard is low in sodium and provides a tasty kick that really makes the egg salad pop. To locate a store near you that carries it, visit www.bookbindersfoods.com or look for a comparable brand at your grocery store.

HARD-COOKED EGGS BY THE DOZEN

Ripped Phase

If you don't use any other tips in this book, use this one. Hard-cooked eggs can be used for many things—eat them plain for a quick protein-packed meal, chop some into a salad, or fancy them up into deviled eggs (see Loaded Eggs on page 110). When I come in from the gym and don't feel like making a protein shake, eggs are the perfect postworkout food. It's easy to pop out the yolks and chow down on a half dozen egg whites in no time flat, then munch a banana and an apple. How easy is that?

12   eggs

HOW TO MAKE IT:

STEP 1   Gently place the eggs in a single layer in a large pot. Cover with cold water by 1".

STEP 2   Over high heat, bring the water to a rolling boil. Cover and reduce the heat to medium-low. Cook for 10 minutes.

STEP 3   Remove from the heat and let sit for 10–15 minutes.

STEP 4   Drain and run cool water into the pot. Remove the cooled eggs and store in the fridge for up to 1 week.

TIP When peeling hard-cooked eggs, use the back of a spoon to crack the shell, then hold the egg under the faucet as you peel it. The water helps wash away the little bits of broken shell.

LOADED EGGS

INGREDIENTS:

12	hard-cooked eggs (see Hard-Cooked Eggs by the Dozen on page 109)
2	tablespoons fat-free plain yogurt
1	tablespoon Dijon mustard
1	teaspoon creamy-style horseradish
	Dash of white pepper
	Dash of smoked or regular paprika

HOW TO MAKE IT:

STEP 1 Cut 8 of the eggs in half and discard the yolks.

STEP 2 In a large bowl, mash the remaining 4 whole eggs with a potato masher until finely mashed. Add the yogurt, mustard, horseradish, and pepper. Mix until creamy.

STEP 3 Spoon 1 tablespoon of the mashed eggs into each egg white half.

STEP 4 Refrigerate for 1 hour.

STEP 5 Sprinkle with paprika.

Makes 4 servings

Per serving: 114 calories, 14 g protein, 2 g carbohydrates, 5 g total fat, 1.5 g saturated fat, 0 g fiber, 239 mg sodium

TIP Use a melon baller to scoop the mashed eggs into the egg white halves.

8

SEAFOOD

Fish is a wonderful source of protein, and it's low in saturated fats and high in the omega-3 fatty acids that can help reduce inflammation, relieve arthritis, prevent heart disease, and increase cognitive brain function. Some of the best Muscle Chow choices include sardines, wild salmon, halibut, mahi mahi, pole-caught or canned light tuna, trap-caught shrimp, farm-raised tilapia, and farmed clams, mussels, and oysters. If you're looking to maintain a lean body with a good set of abs, you need to add some of the recipes that follow to your weekly regimen.

Whatever type of fish you choose, be sure it doesn't smell fishy. If it does—even if the fishmonger tells you he flew it in last night—you don't want it stinking up your house. Fresh fish should have a pleasant, appetizing, briny sea smell. If it doesn't look or smell appetizing, opt for beef or poultry instead and try again next week.

As a general rule, fish should be cooked for 8 to 10 minutes per inch of thickness, measured at the thickest portion. When baking fish, it's a good idea to fold under any thin, tapered edges to create more thickness and even cooking.

QUICK-BAKE FISH

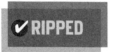 **RIPPED**

The types of fish recommended in this recipe are slightly firm and perfect for breading and baking. If your favorite isn't listed, feel free to substitute it in this recipe.

INGREDIENTS:

½   teaspoon extra-virgin olive oil

2   tilapia, grouper, cod, haddock, halibut, or snapper fillets (6 ounces each), rinsed and dried

1   cup 4C® Carb Careful Plain Breadcrumbs

¼   teaspoon smoked or regular paprika

½   teaspoon McCormick's Salt Free All-Purpose Seasoning

       Pinch of ground black pepper

½   lemon

HOW TO MAKE IT:

STEP 1 Preheat the oven to 450°F. Pour the oil into a shallow baking dish and swirl the dish to coat it with oil. Wipe the excess oil with a paper towel. Lay the fillets in the dish side by side about ¼" apart.

STEP 2 In a bowl, mix together the bread crumbs, paprika, all-purpose seasoning, and pepper. Sprinkle an even layer of the crumb mix over the fillets.

STEP 3 Squeeze the juice of the lemon over both fillets.

STEP 4 Bake for 8 to 10 minutes. Raise the oven temperature to broil and broil for 1 to 2 minutes, or until the crumbs start to brown and the fish flakes easily.

Makes 2 servings

Per serving: 322 calories, 56 g protein, 16 g carbohydrates, 2 g total fat, 0.5 g saturated fat, 8 g fiber, 100 mg sodium

SERVING SUGGESTION: This is excellent served with the Classic Steamed Veggies on page 154, the Baked Asparagus with Sea Salt on page 161, or the Oven-Roasted Zucchini on page 162. All of these sides offer nutritious carbs with healthy fiber to help balance out the nutritional profile of the meal—plus they enhance the taste of the dish.

TIP Use a knife to check the fish for doneness. Simply insert the point and twist. This allows you to see into the fillet without breaking it apart. It should look opaque and flake easily.

POACHED SALMON WITH STEAMED VEGGIES

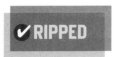

This easy-to-make meal is a fast way to get protein, glutamine, creatine, phyto-nutrients, and a healthy dose of essential fatty acids in your diet.

INGREDIENTS:

1   (6-ounce) salmon fillet (see tip)

½   cup chopped celery

        Pinch of lemon-dill seasoning

        Pinch of ground black pepper

PICK 3 VEGGIES FROM THIS LIST:

10   to 12 asparagus spears, bottoms cut off

2   yellow squash, sliced

1   zucchini, sliced

1   cup yellow or green beans, trimmed

1   cup Brussels sprouts

1   cup snow peas

1   cup sliced mushrooms

½   cup broccoli florets

NOTE Don't let the high fat content of this dish scare you. Remember, salmon is loaded with essential fatty acids—the good fat!

HOW TO MAKE IT:

STEP 1 Place the salmon in a deep skillet. Add enough water to cover the salmon by 1".

STEP 2 Add the celery, lemon-dill seasoning, and pepper. Bring to a slow boil over medium heat. Cook for 10 to 15 minutes, or until the salmon is opaque at the thickest point. Use a knife to check for doneness—insert the point and twist to make sure the fillet is light pink all the way through.

STEP 3 Remove to a plate. Lightly scrape off the skin and fat line.

STEP 4 Place a steamer basket in a large pot with 2" of water. Bring to a boil over high heat. Place your choice of 3 veggies in the basket and steam for 3 to 5 minutes, or until crisp-tender.

Makes 1 serving

Per serving: 404 calories, 42 g protein, 18 g carbohydrates, 19 g total fat, 4 g saturated fat, 7 g fiber, 160 mg sodium

EASY ROASTED SALMON

INGREDIENTS:

4	salmon fillets (6 ounces each)
1	teaspoon balsamic vinegar
¼	cup 4C® Carb Careful Plain Breadcrumbs
2	lemons
¼	teaspoon ground black pepper
2	tablespoons chopped dried or fresh parsley
4	small yellow squash, halved
1	tablespoon grated Parmesan cheese

NOTE Don't let the high fat content of this dish scare you. Remember, salmon is loaded with essential fatty acids—the good fat!

HOW TO MAKE IT:

STEP 1 Preheat the oven to 400°F. Place the salmon on a broiling rack. Drizzle with the balsamic vinegar. Sprinkle 2 tablespoons of the bread crumbs over the fillets. Squeeze the juice of 1 lemon over the top. Sprinkle with half the pepper and 1 tablespoon of the parsley. Thinly slice the remaining lemon and place a slice on top of each fillet.

STEP 2 Lay the squash halves cut sides up around the salmon. In a small bowl, mix the cheese with the remaining bread crumbs, pepper, and parsley. Sprinkle the crumb mixture over the squash.

STEP 3 Bake for 15 to 20 minutes, or until the salmon is opaque and the squash is slightly tender.

Makes 4 servings

Per serving: 364 calories, 39 g protein, 8 g carbohydrates, 19 g total fat, 4 g saturated fat, 2 g fiber, 124 mg sodium

TIP There's more than one way to skin a salmon. You can hack off the skin while the fish is still raw, or you can use a spatula to gently scrape away the skin once the fish has cooked. The second way is much easier. Be sure to also scrape the fat line (the gray fatty stuff) from under the fillet as well. If you don't, the salmon will taste and smell fishy.

BAMBOO-STEAMED FISH AND VEGGIES

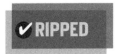

This dish requires a round, two-tier 10" bamboo steamer, a piece of equipment you can find at any store that carries a wide range of cookware. (I picked mine up at the local mall). The stackable tiers allow you to cook a few different foods at the same time. Be sure to get a pan that fits your 10" bamboo steamer. The steamer should fit snugly into the pan, with a little room around the edges to keep water and steam condensation from dripping onto the stove top and creating a mess. The best thing to do is to buy both the pan and the steamer together to ensure a proper fit.

INGREDIENTS:

2	large lettuce leaves
2	red snapper fillets (6 ounces each), skinned
1	tablespoon chopped fresh dill
	Pinch of ground black pepper
½	lemon, thinly sliced into 4 slices
15	grape or cherry tomatoes
2	cups broccoli florets
	No-salt lemon-pepper seasoning

HOW TO MAKE IT:

STEP 1 Fan the lettuce out in the lowest tier of a bamboo steamer. Place a fillet on top of each leaf. Sprinkle with the dill and pepper. Top each fillet with 2 of the lemon slices.

STEP 2 Place the tomatoes and broccoli in the upper tier of the steamer. Sprinkle with the lemon-pepper seasoning (to taste). Place the upper steamer tier atop the lower tier and cover with the lid.

STEP 3 Pour 1" to 1½" of water into the pan that fits the steamer. Place the steamer in the pan, making sure the water touches the bottom edge of the steamer to create a nice seal. Bring to a boil over medium-high heat. Steam for 15 minutes, or until the fish flakes easily.

Makes 2 servings

Per serving: 220 calories, 38 g protein, 10 g carbohydrates, 3 g total fat, 0.5 g saturated fat, 4 g fiber, 148 mg sodium

ALMOND-CRUSTED TILAPIA

INGREDIENTS:

2	tilapia fillets (6 ounces each), rinsed and dried
2	tablespoons unbleached or all-purpose flour
2	egg whites
	Juice of ½ lemon
20	unsalted roasted almonds, crushed
¼	cup 4C Carb Careful Plain Breadcrumbs
½	teaspoon chopped dried or fresh parsley
	Pinch of ground black pepper

HOW TO MAKE IT:

STEP 1 Preheat the oven to 350°F.

STEP 2 Put the flour in a shallow dish.

STEP 3 In another shallow dish, mix together the egg whites and lemon juice.

STEP 4 In a third shallow dish, mix together the almonds, bread crumbs, parsley, and pepper.

STEP 5 Dredge the fish first in the flour, then in the egg mixture, and then in the crumb mixture.

STEP 6 Place the fish in a shallow baking dish. Sprinkle with any remaining crumb mixture. Bake for 15 minutes. Raise the oven temperature to broil and broil for 1 to 2 minutes, or until browned (watch carefully so as not to burn).

Makes 2 servings

Per serving: 464 calories, 53 g protein, 18 g carbohydrates, 21 g total fat, 2.5 g saturated fat, 6 g fiber, 157 mg sodium

TIP To crush the almonds, put them between two paper plates, then roll a wine bottle over the plates until all the almonds are crunched into pieces. You'll notice that this recipe is relatively high in fat. That's because almonds contain heart-healthy monounsaturated fats. They're also high in fiber.

FIX 'N' EAT SARDINE SANDY

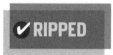 RIPPED

INGREDIENTS:

1   can (3.75 ounces) low-sodium sardines packed in water, drained, rinsed, and patted dry

2   slices Ezekiel 4:9 Organic Sprouted 100% Whole Grain Flourless Low Sodium Bread

      Honey mustard (use the lowest-sodium one you can find)

HOW TO MAKE IT:

STEP 1 Lay the sardines on 1 slice of bread.

STEP 2 Add the honey mustard (to taste).

STEP 3 Top with the other slice of bread.

Makes 1 serving

Per serving: 401 calories, 23 g protein, 37 g carbohydrates, 5.5 g total fat, 1 g saturated fat, 7 g fiber, 35 mg sodium

SWEET TUNA SALAD IN ROMAINE BOATS

Whether friends stop by or you just want a lazy-Sunday-watching-football lunch, these are simple to make and will go in a hurry. The sweet taste of the fruit complements the tuna and helps keep it moist.

INGREDIENTS:

1	can (4 ounces) low-sodium chunk white tuna packed in water, drained and rinsed
1	hard-cooked egg, chopped
½	pear, chopped
2	heaping tablespoons fat-free sour cream
1	heaping tablespoon dried cranberries
2	teaspoons lemon juice
4	medium leaves Romaine lettuce
2	tablespoons sunflower seeds
1	apple, cut into wedges

HOW TO MAKE IT:

STEP 1 Put the tuna in a large bowl and break it apart with a fork. Mix in the egg, pear, sour cream, cranberries, and lemon juice.

STEP 2 Spoon one-fourth of the tuna salad onto each lettuce leaf.

STEP 3 Sprinkle each serving with ½ tablespoon sunflower seeds. Garnish with the apple wedges.

Makes 4 servings

Per serving: 135 calories, 10 g protein, 14 g carbohydrates, 5 g total fat, 1 g saturated fat, 2.5 g fiber, 36 mg sodium

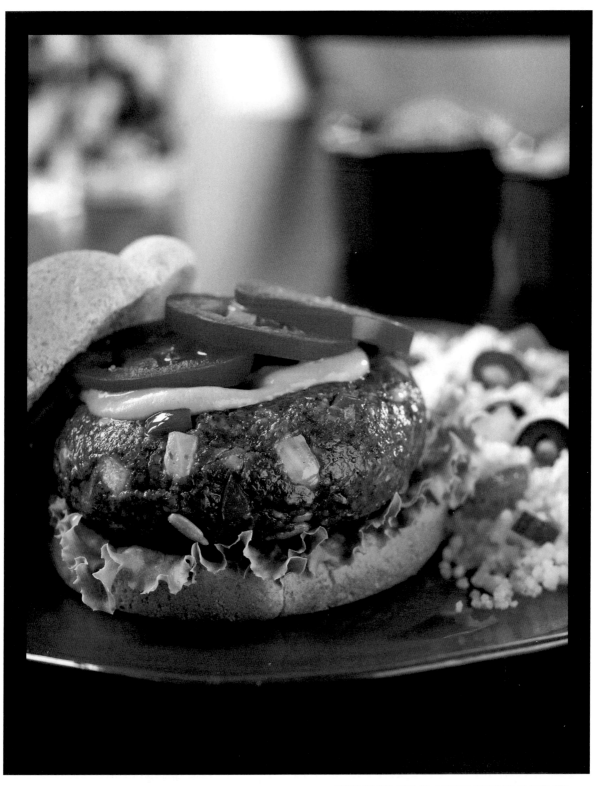

POWER BURGER, PAGE 59; BASIC COUSCOUS SALAD, PAGE 144

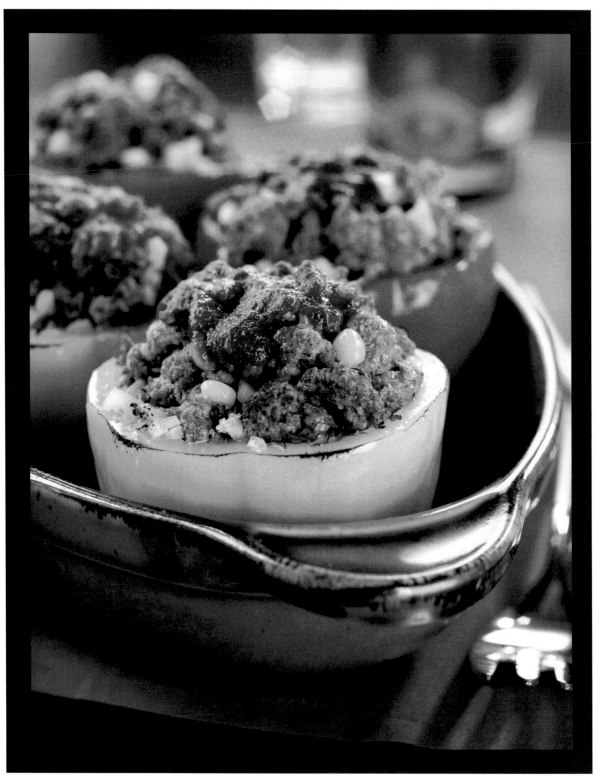

BEEF BOMBS, PAGE 63

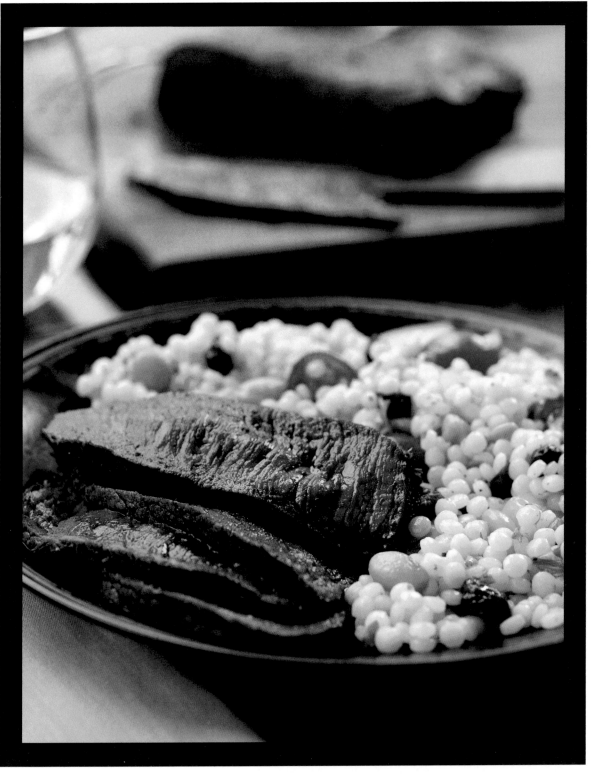

LONDON BROIL, PAGE 65; VEGETABLE-PACKED ISRAELI COUSCOUS, PAGE 145

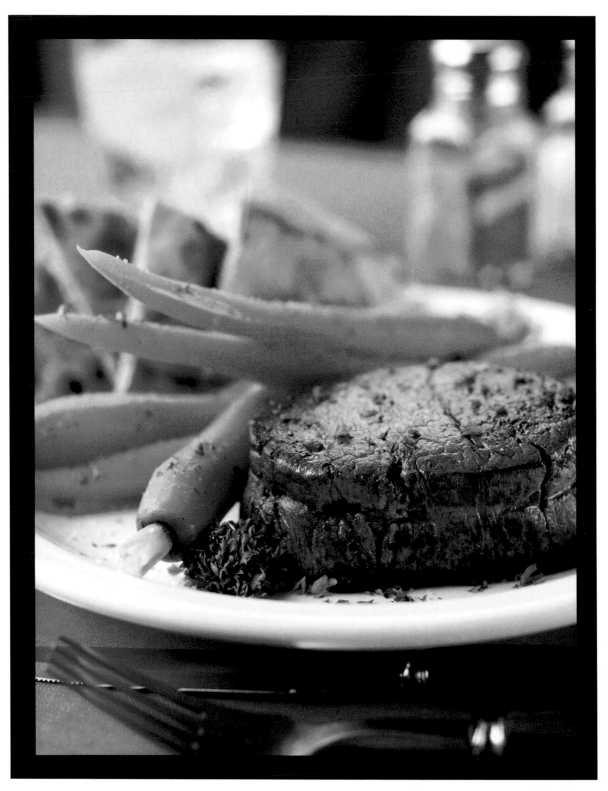

FILET WITH ROASTED CARROTS, PAGE 66

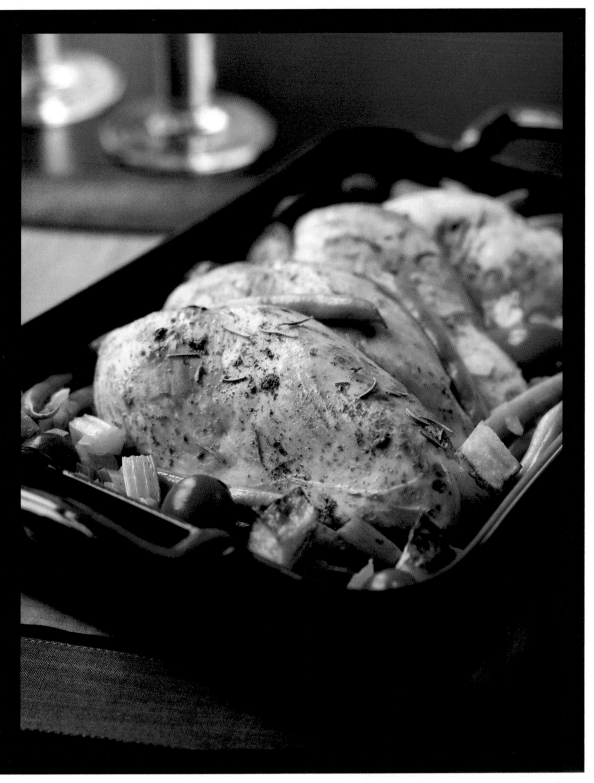

ROSEMARY CHICKEN WITH ROASTED VEGETABLES, PAGE 83

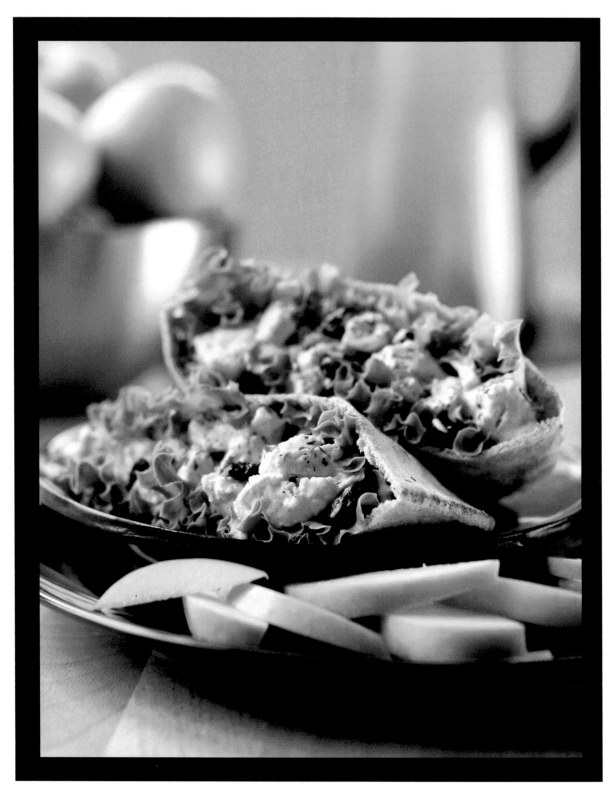

2-MINUTE CHICKEN SALAD PITA, PAGE 73

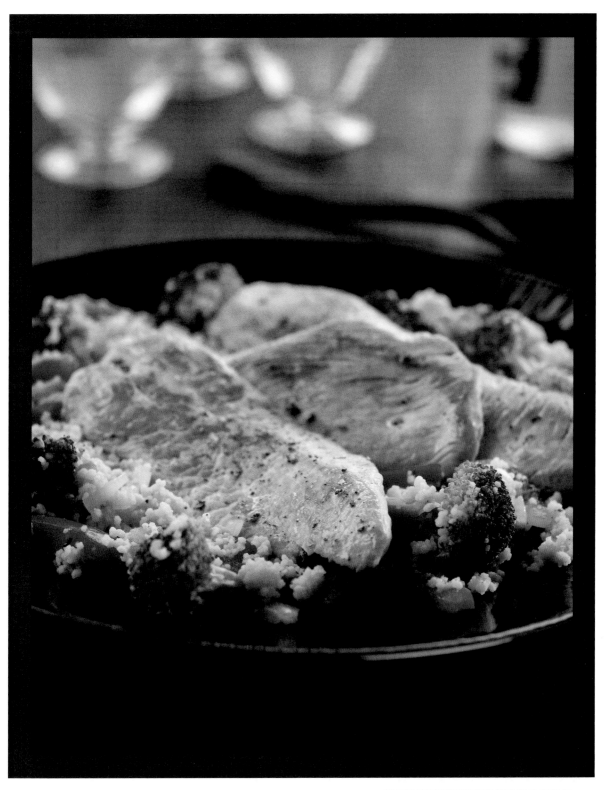

TURKEY AND BROCCOLI WITH COUSCOUS, PAGE 94

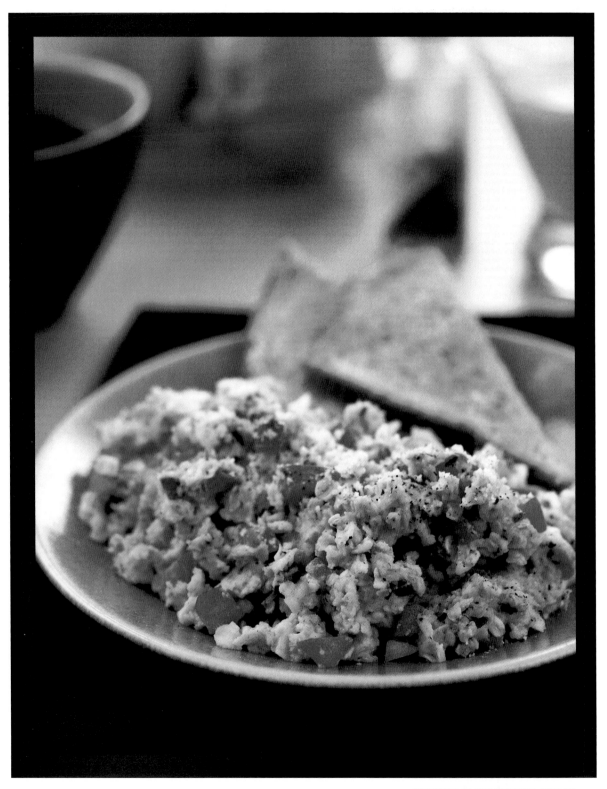

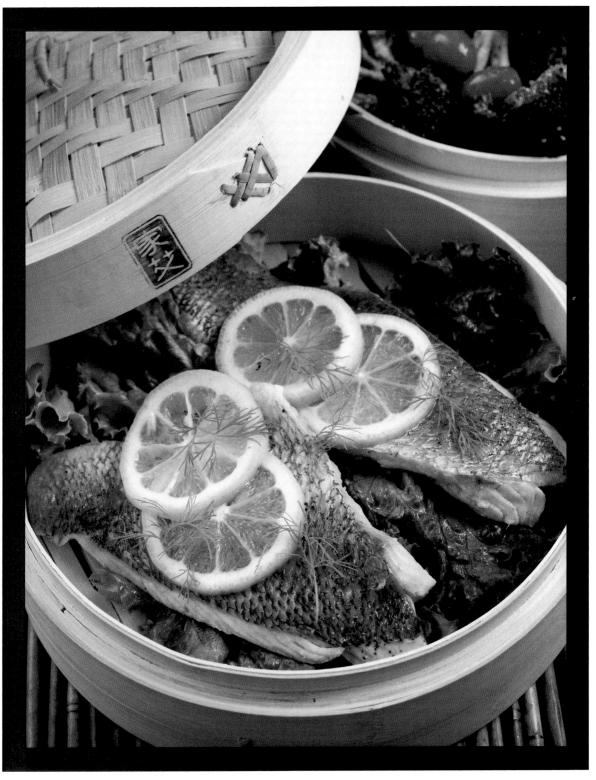

BAMBOO-STEAMED FISH AND VEGGIES, PAGE 115

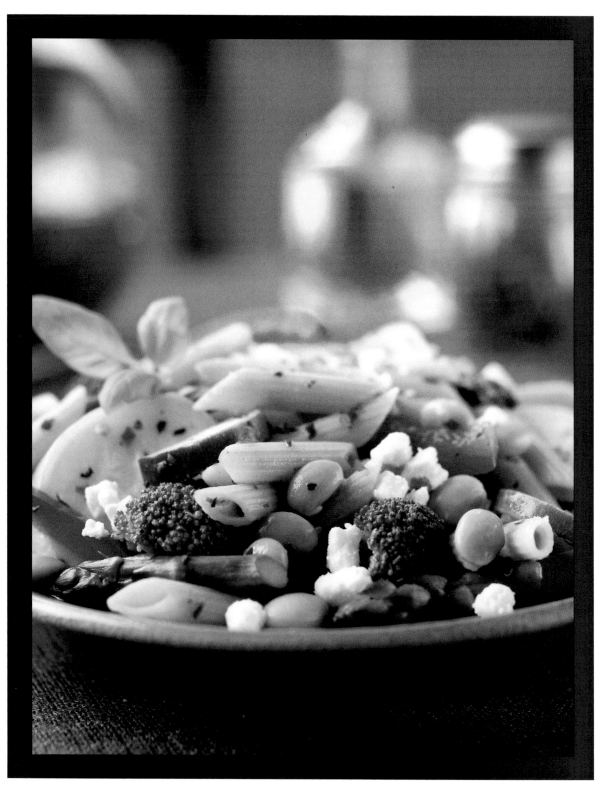

ULTIMATE POWER PASTA, PAGE 131

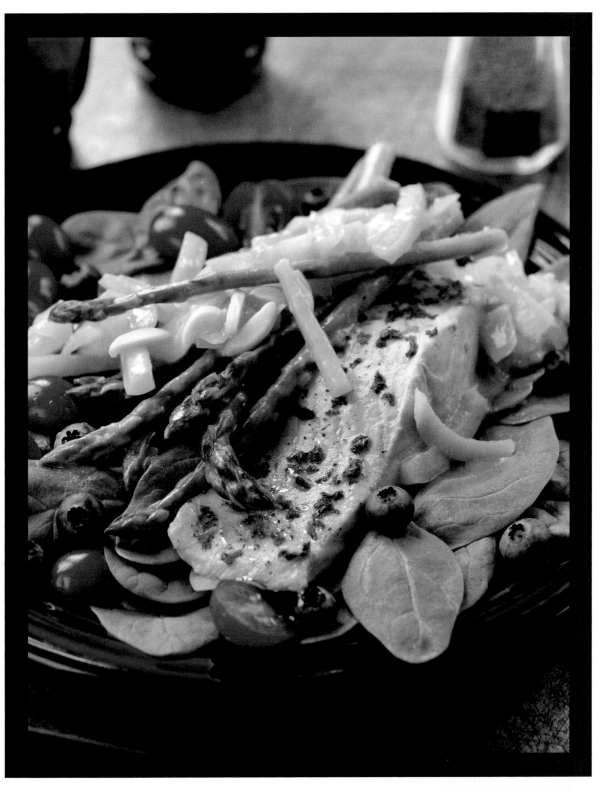

LOADED SPINACH SALAD, PAGE 174

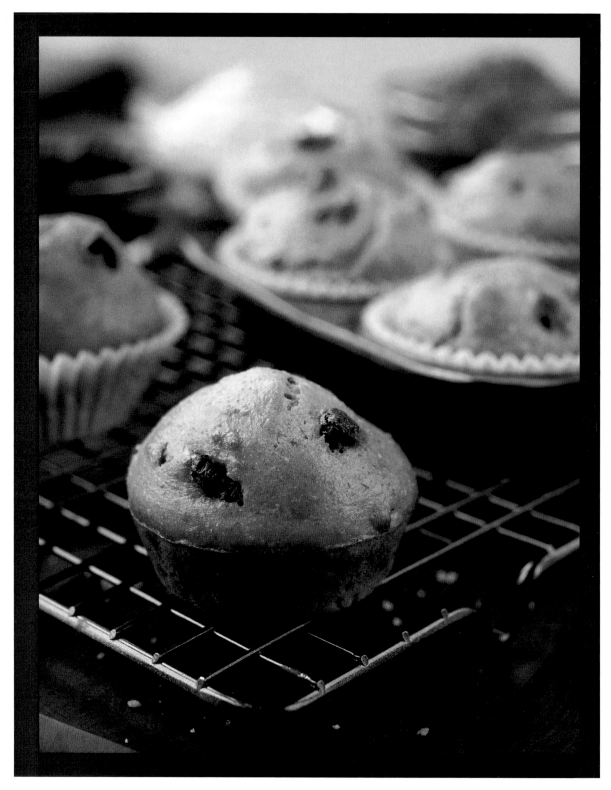

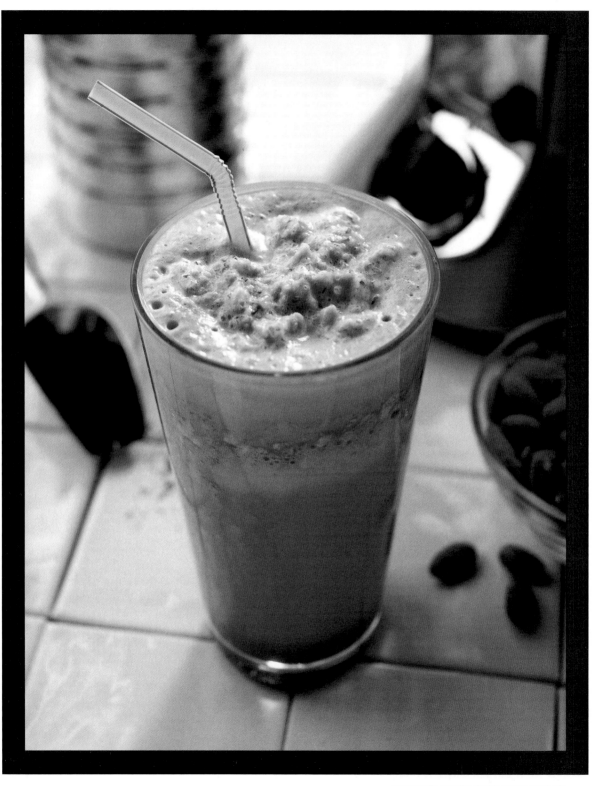

CHOCOLATE ALMOND MOCHA BLAST, PAGE 198

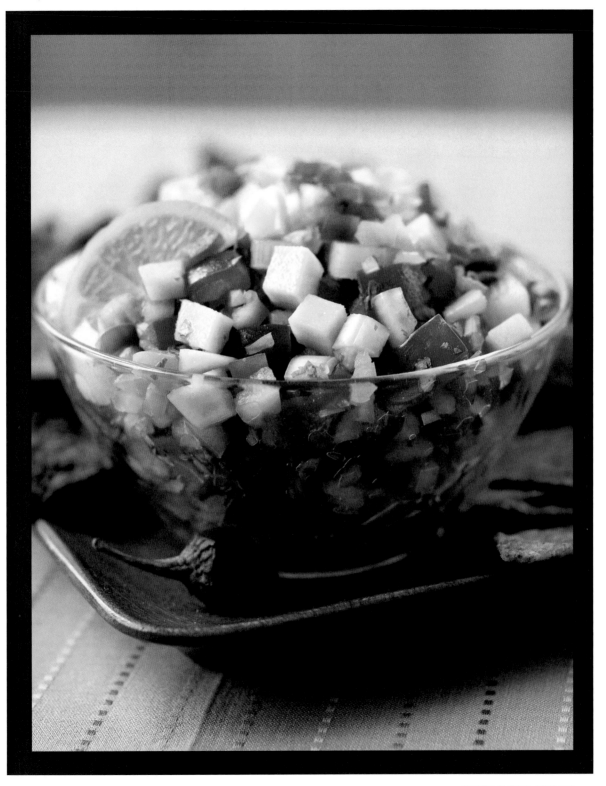

METABOLIC SALSA, PAGE 223

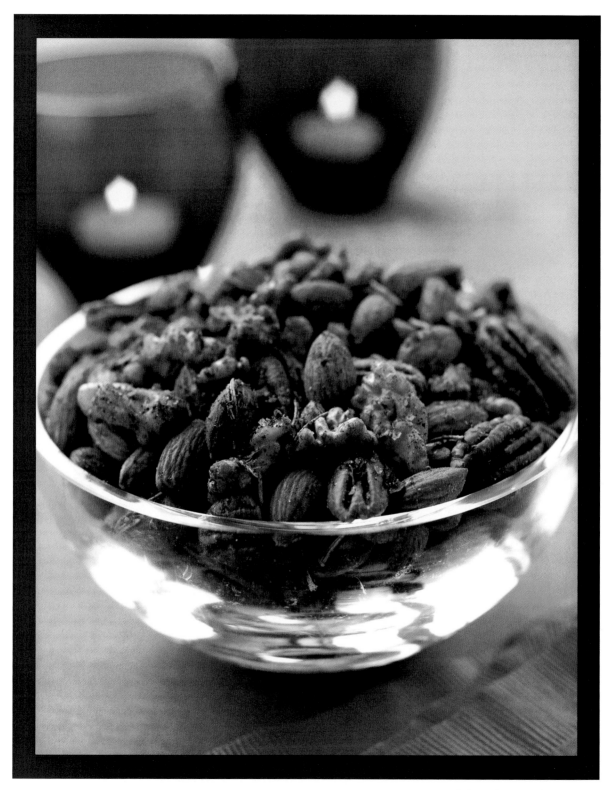

SPICY ROASTED NUTS, PAGE 229

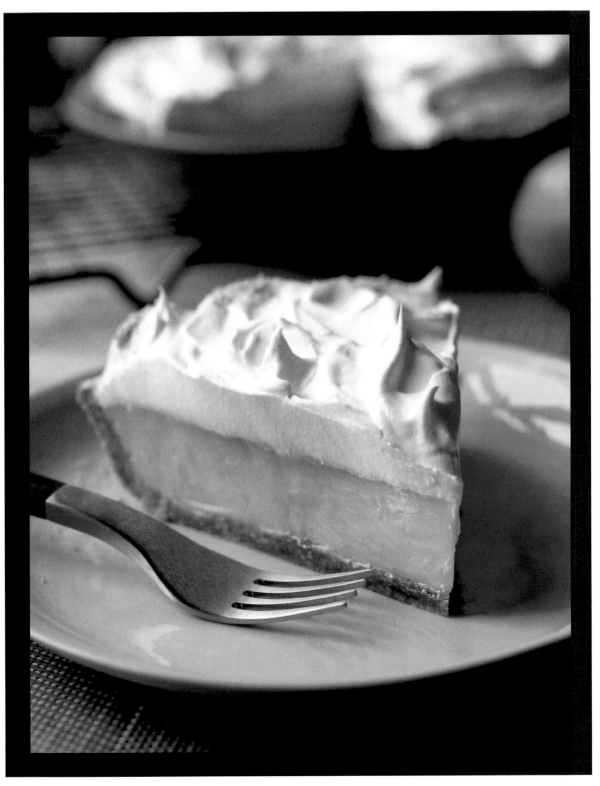

KEY LIME PIE, PAGE 240

QUICK ROTINI 'N' CLAMS

Once you learn how to make this dish, you'll find that it's super quick and easy. The asparagus adds a nice flavor and precludes the need for a separate vegetable side dish.

INGREDIENTS:

1	**heaping cup rotini**
½	**teaspoon extra-virgin olive oil**
½	**small yellow onion, chopped**
1	**teaspoon minced garlic**
	Pinch of black pepper
15	**littleneck clams, washed well (see note)**
15	**asparagus spears, with bottoms cut off, chopped**
1	**can (8 ounces) no-salt tomato sauce**
¼	**cup water, at room temperature (see note)**
1	**tablespoon chopped dried or fresh parsley**

HOW TO MAKE IT:

STEP 1 Cook the rotini according to the package directions. Drain and set aside.

STEP 2 In a large saucepan, add the oil and heat over medium-high heat. Add the onion, garlic, and pepper. Cook for 1 minute.

STEP 3 Reduce the heat to medium-low. Add the clams, asparagus, tomato sauce, and water. Stir and cover. Cook for 5 to 6 minutes. The clams will begin to open after about 2 minutes and should take no longer than 6 minutes. Throw away any that haven't opened by that point.

STEP 4 Ladle half of the clam sauce over ½ cup of the pasta. Sprinkle with the parsley.

Makes 2 servings

Per serving: 219 calories, 16 g protein, 33 g carbohydrates, 2.5 g total fat, 0.5 g saturated fat, 6 g fiber, 57 mg sodium

NOTE Before cooking clams, discard any that are not tightly shut. It's important to make sure the water is tepid, because you don't want to interrupt the cooking process by adding cold water.

FLEX YOUR MUSSELS

Mussels are the original fast food. Seriously—they cook in about 3 minutes. Before you begin, rinse them well and look them over. Discard any with open shells. They should all be tightly shut before you add them to the pot.

INGREDIENTS:

2	ribs celery, chopped
1	small yellow onion, chopped
½	cup water
½	teaspoon extra-virgin olive oil
½	teaspoon McCormick Salt Free All-Purpose Seasoning
	Pinch of ground black pepper
2	pounds mussels, washed well
1	cup dry white wine
2	tablespoons chopped dried or fresh parsley

HOW TO MAKE IT:

STEP 1 In a large pot, combine the celery, onion, water, oil, all-purpose seasoning, and pepper. Bring to a boil over high heat.

STEP 2 Add the mussels, wine, and parsley. Reduce the heat to medium. Cover.

STEP 3 Cook for 2 to 3 minutes, or until the mussels have opened. Discard any that haven't opened.

Makes 2 servings

Per serving: 310 calories, 24 g protein, 16 g carbohydrates, 5.5 g total fat, 1 g saturated fat, 2 g fiber, 610 mg sodium

SERVING SUGGESTION: Give garlic bread a Muscle Chow makeover. Simply brush a small amount of olive oil onto whole grain bread; sprinkle with some ground black pepper, a little minced garlic, and a pinch of parsley; and toast to a golden brown.

TIP When mussels are harvested, a little salt water gets trapped inside. When you cook them, they open and that briny water is released into the dish. This isn't a bad thing, but it does raise the overall sodium content of the meal.

SWORDFISH ON THE GRILL

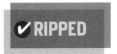

The first time I had grilled swordfish was in the Canary Islands. After spending a lot of time in the islands because of my career, I learned to absolutely love this clean, easily grilled fish.

INGREDIENTS:

2   swordfish steaks (each about 6 ounces and ½" thick), rinsed and dried

1   teaspoon extra-virgin olive oil

1   teaspoon no-salt lemon-pepper seasoning

HOW TO MAKE IT:

STEP 1 Coat a grill rack with cooking spray. Preheat the grill to medium-low.

STEP 2 Lightly brush the swordfish with the oil. Sprinkle ½ teaspoon of the lemon-pepper seasoning on one side. Place the swordfish seasoned side down on the grill. Cook for 5 to 6 minutes.

STEP 3 Sprinkle the remaining ½ teaspoon lemon-pepper seasoning on the fish. Flip. Grill for 5 minutes, or until the fish flakes easily.

Makes 2 servings

Per serving: 227 calories, 34 g protein, 0 g carbohydrates, 9 g total fat, 2 g saturated fat, 0 g fiber, 173 mg sodium

TIP Even though swordfish will hold together much better than other fish, as a rule you don't want to flip fish more than one time.

RIPPED TIP
If you're preparing this dish during a Ripped Phase, omit the olive oil to help cut down the fat content.

GRILLED AHI TUNA AND VEGETABLES

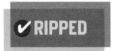 **RIPPED**

This entire meal cooks completely on the grill, so you can hang outside with an iced tea in one hand and a spatula in the other, just grillin' and chillin'. Twenty minutes from beginning to end.

INGREDIENTS:

¼   **cup extra-virgin olive oil**

       Pinch of ground black pepper

15   **asparagus spears, with bottoms cut off**

2   **plum tomatoes, halved**

1   **medium eggplant, halved**

       No-salt lemon-pepper seasoning

2   **sushi-grade tuna fillets (6 to 8 ounces each)**

HOW TO MAKE IT:

STEP 1 Coat the grill rack with cooking spray. Preheat the grill to medium.

STEP 2 In a small bowl, mix together the oil and black pepper. Brush a light coat onto the asparagus, tomatoes, and eggplant.

STEP 3 Sprinkle the vegetables and tuna with the lemon-pepper seasoning (to taste).

STEP 4 Grill the veggies and tuna in the following order:

- Lay the eggplant cut side down on the grill (they will grill for around 16 minutes).

- After 3 minutes, lay the tuna fillets on the grill (they will grill for 10 minutes).

- After 5 minutes, lay the tomatoes cut side down. Sprinkle everything with a little more lemon-pepper seasoning.

- After the eggplant has been cooking for 10 minutes and the tomatoes for 3 minutes, flip both.

- After another 3 minutes, flip the tuna, add the asparagus, and remove the tomatoes.

- After another 3 minutes, remove the asparagus and the tuna. The eggplant should be tender, but if not, grill for a few more minutes.

STEP 5 Serve each tuna fillet with half of the veggies.

Makes 2 servings

Per serving: 405 calories, 46 g protein, 23 g carbohydrates, 16 g total fat, 2.5 g saturated fat, 13 g fiber, 74 mg sodium

RIPPED TIP
If you're preparing this dish in a Ripped Phase, substitute olive oil cooking spray for the ¼ cup olive oil. Just spray right on the veggies and grill as directed.

GRILLED TUNA WITH PEANUT SAUCE

This is a simple way to prepare fresh tuna fillets, and the prep time takes only minutes. Be sure you get fresh, nice-looking tuna without dark spots. I often buy sushi-grade tuna, which is best cooked medium-rare.

INGREDIENTS:

4	**tuna steaks (each 6 ounces and 1" thick)**
2	**teaspoons extra-virgin olive oil**
	Fresh ground black pepper
3	**tablespoons natural peanut butter**
2	**tablespoons water**
	Juice of ½ lemon
1	**tablespoon balsamic vinegar**
1	**heaping teaspoon brown sugar**

HOW TO MAKE IT:

STEP 1 Preheat the grill to medium. Brush the tuna with the oil. Lightly season with the pepper (to taste). Grill for 7 to 10 minutes on each side, or until the fish is just opaque.

STEP 2 In a microwaveable bowl, combine the peanut butter, water, lemon juice, balsamic vinegar, and brown sugar. Microwave on high for 30 seconds. Mix well.

STEP 3 Divide the sauce evenly among the tuna fillets.

Makes 4 servings

Per serving: 350 calories, 42 g protein, 5 g carbohydrates, 16.5 g total fat, 3 g saturated fat, 1 g fiber, 113.5 mg sodium

SERVING SUGGESTION: Add side dishes of wild rice (prepared according to the package directions) and a small salad of mixed greens. One of my favorite rice blends is Countrywild by Lundberg. The company offers a few other variations that are super flavorful and aromatic.

NOTE If you're concerned with fat (even though peanut butter contains healthy monounsaturated fat), reduce the amount of peanut butter to 1 tablespoon. You can prepare the peanut sauce ahead of time, but you'll want to microwave it just before serving the fish.

FOOLPROOF GRILLED FISH PACKETS

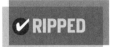

Fish can easily become dry or chewy when it's overcooked. That's where aluminum foil cooking packets come in handy—they seal in moisture throughout the cooking process, which takes just 15 minutes. I've listed some of the fish I enjoy the most because of their flavor and versatility. Salmon is my personal favorite. If your favorite isn't included, feel free to sub it into this recipe. You can make multiple packets to match the number of mouths you're feeding and cook them on the grill all at the same time.

INGREDIENTS:

1   salmon, grouper, tilapia, or snapper fillet (6 ounces), rinsed and dried

       Pinch of no-salt lemon-pepper seasoning

HOW TO MAKE IT:

STEP 1 Preheat the grill to medium. Tear off two 14" pieces of aluminum foil. (I like the new nonstick foil.)

STEP 2 Lay the fish in the center of one foil sheet and sprinkle with the lemon-pepper seasoning.

STEP 3 Cover with the second foil sheet and tightly fold the edges together with two ½" folds on each side to seal completely. (Do a final half-fold upward so no liquid leaks out.)

STEP 4 Grill for 10 minutes. The packet will expand as it fills with steam. Rotate a half turn and grill for 5 minutes longer.

STEP 5 Cut an × in the middle of the packet, pull back the cut edges, and dish out onto a plate. The fish should be opaque and flake easily.

Makes 1 serving

Per serving: 311 calories, 34 g protein, 0 g carbohydrates, 18.5 g total fat, 4 g saturated fat, 0 g fiber, 128 mg sodium

SERVING SUGGESTION: Because this dish provides zero carbs, you can also throw some zucchini and yellow squash onto the grill to cook at the same time as the fish. Just cut the veggies in half lengthwise, brush with a little olive oil, and sprinkle on a little ground black pepper. Grill cut side down for 4 minutes, then flip and grill for 4 minutes longer.

GRILLED SALMON BULGUR PACKETS

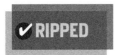 **RIPPED**

I like to use bulgur wheat for its whole grain goodness, high fiber, and low sodium content, but you can also substitute instant brown rice. Even though the recipe calls for yellow squash, feel free to get creative with your veggies. Carrots, zucchini, green peas, and broccoli also work well with this dish.

INGREDIENTS:

¾   **cup boiling water**

½   **cup bulgur wheat**

1   **salmon fillet (6 ounces), skinned**

1   **medium yellow squash, chopped**

½   **lemon**

           Pinch of no-salt lemon-pepper seasoning

HOW TO MAKE IT:

STEP 1 In a large bowl, pour the water over the bulgur. Stir, cover with plastic wrap, and let sit for 15 minutes, or until almost all of the water has been absorbed.

STEP 2 Preheat the grill to medium. Tear off two 14" pieces of aluminum foil. (I like the new nonstick foil.) Lay the salmon in the center of one foil sheet and pour the bulgur around it. Add the squash around the fish, squeeze the lemon over the top, and sprinkle with the lemon-pepper seasoning.

STEP 3 Cover with the second foil sheet, and tightly fold the edges together with two ½" folds on each side to seal completely. (Do a final half-fold upward so no liquid leaks out.)

STEP 4 Grill for 10 minutes. The packet will expand as it fills with steam. Rotate a half turn and grill for 5 minutes longer.

STEP 5 Cut an × in the middle of the foil packet, pull back the cut edges, and dish out onto a plate. The fish should be opaque.

Makes 1 serving

Per serving: 585 calories, 44 g protein, 61 g carbohydrates, 19 g total fat, 4 g saturated fat, 16 g fiber, 144 mg sodium

RIPPED TIP

Even though salmon is chock full of heart healthy omega-3 fatty acids, when in a Ripped Phase it's best to limit this oily fish to once or twice a week.

SHRIMP KEBABS WITH GRILLED CORN

This is a great dish for a get-together. It sounds like a lot of work and does take some prep time, but the actual grilling time is about 20 minutes. I like to serve this with a big mixed salad and a bowl of cut-up mango, peaches, blueberries, and raspberries. When the meal all comes together, it's clean, healthy food full of rich textures, colors, and flavors.

INGREDIENTS:

4	ears corn, with husks intact
1	pound shrimp, shelled and deveined (keep the tails on for more flavor)
1	tablespoon extra-virgin olive oil
	No-salt lemon-pepper seasoning
1	orange or yellow bell pepper, seeded and cut into chunks
2	lemons, cut into wedges
1	pint cherry or grape tomatoes
1	large sweet onion, quartered
	Ground black pepper

HOW TO MAKE IT:

STEP 1 Soak 25 wooden skewers in water for 30 minutes. This will keep the skewers from burning on the grill.

STEP 2 Soak the corn in a large pot of water at room temperature for 15 to 20 minutes. This will keep the husks from burning on the grill.

STEP 3 Preheat the grill to medium-low.

STEP 4 Skewer the shrimp through the thick upper portion and into the thinner lower portion. This will help them lay flat on the grill. Leave a little space between shrimp, and fill as many skewers as you need. (One pound of shrimp should yield 8 to 10 skewers.) Brush with 1 teaspoon of the oil. Sprinkle with the lemon-pepper seasoning (to taste).

STEP 5 Evenly divide the bell pepper, lemons, tomatoes, and onion among the remaining skewers, alternating the veggies. Lightly brush with 1 teaspoon of the oil. Sprinkle with the lemon-pepper seasoning (to taste).

STEP 6 Carefully peel back the corn husks without tearing them off completely. Remove the silk and discard. Lightly brush the ears with the remaining 1 teaspoon oil and sprinkle with the black pepper (to taste). Close the husks around the ears. Tie the top of each husk with kitchen twine. Clip any excess twine so it doesn't hang down into the grill and catch fire.

STEP 7 Place the corn on the grill. After about 5 minutes, add the veggie skewers. Turn the corn and veggies frequently to make sure they're cooked on all sides and browned nicely. After 10 to 15 minutes longer, raise the grill temperature to medium. Cut the twine on the corn husks, peel back the husks (you can leave them on for a rustic look), and continue to grill the ears, turning, until the kernels are slightly brown. Add the shrimp skewers. Grill for 4 to 6 minutes, turning as they char.

Makes 4 servings

Per serving: 261 calories, 26 g protein, 25 g carbohydrates, 8 g total fat, 1 g saturated fat, 4 g fiber, 160 mg sodium

SERVING SUGGESTION: If you're serving more than four people, cut the corn from the cob over a large serving bowl, then slide the veggies off the skewers and into the bowl, setting aside the lemon wedges. Add ½ cup chopped cilantro and ground black pepper to taste. Squeeze the juice of ½ lemon over it, toss, and serve as a side dish garnished with a few of the reserved lemon wedges. Serve the shrimp skewers on a serving plate.

MAHI FISH WRAPS

INGREDIENTS:

4   mahi mahi fillets (6 ounces each)

1   teaspoon extra-virgin olive oil

         No-salt lemon-pepper seasoning

1   cup fat-free plain yogurt

         Juice of 2 limes

         Ground black pepper

8   large leaves Boston lettuce

2   tomatoes, chopped

1   cucumber, seeded and grated

1   avocado, chopped

1   cup bean sprouts

1   cup shredded carrots

HOW TO MAKE IT:

STEP 1 Coat a grill rack with cooking spray. Preheat the grill to medium.

STEP 2 Brush the fish with the oil. Sprinkle with the lemon-pepper seasoning (to taste).

STEP 3 Grill the fish for 6 minutes on each side, flipping once, or until the fish flakes easily.

STEP 4 In a bowl, mix together the yogurt, lime juice, and pepper (to taste).

STEP 5 Fill each lettuce leaf with about 2 tablespoons each of the tomatoes, cucumber, avocado, sprouts, and carrots. Top each with several chunks of mahi mahi. Drizzle each with an equal amount of the yogurt sauce. Fold each lettuce leaf into a wrap.

Makes 4 servings

Per serving (2 wraps): 293 calories, 37 g protein, 18 g carbohydrates, 9 g total fat, 1.5 g saturated fat, 6 g fiber, 213 mg sodium

VARIATION: Go sweet with this dish. Instead of the cucumber, avocado, sprouts, and carrots, use mango, pineapple, and cilantro.

9

PASTAS & GRAINS

Carbohydrates are a main energy source for your body and your brain. They help give you an overall sense of well-being, and they supply fuel that is stored in your liver and muscles. I believe that higher-carb/lower-carb days are extremely important when it comes to achieving strides in and out of the gym—from muscle building to strength, size, and especially getting lean. This balance can be called carb-shifting, and that's where pasta and grains come in handy. When trying to saturate my system with an abundance of long-lasting, low-fat carbs, the best carbohydrate-rich foods I can think of are pasta and grains. Let me explain.

When I string together several lower-carb days in a row by eating lots of protein along with fibrous vegetables and moderate fruits and grains, I notice that my muscles begin to look a little flat. This is due to a lack of glycogen. Because glycogen is stored via water, it increases muscle volume. When your muscles lack glycogen, they have less volume. Think of a water balloon that's empty and deflated versus one that's been filled at the faucet till it's big, round, and firm. When I chow complex carbohydrates (like pasta or whole grain rice)—especially after three to four days of not eating them—I feel it the next day in the gym. I have more energy and motivation, I'm stronger, and I can achieve a fuller pump during my workout. And because superficial veins are located close to the surface of the skin, an increase of cell volume within the muscle pushes those veins to the surface. That means more vascularity—something many guys strive for from an aesthetic point of view. It can also be an indicator of how lean you're getting, because more visible vascularity means less body fat between the skin and the muscle.

Let's quickly talk about how carb-shifting (higher-carb/lower-carb days) can also make you leaner. As I talked about earlier in the book, it's important to consume food every two to three hours. This helps fuel your body on a consistent basis, signaling your body to liberate calories and keep your metabolism revved. When you don't eat for extended periods of time, it's just the opposite—your metabolism slows down to preserve calories. By utilizing the method of carb-shifting, you take this concept to the next level by keeping your body off guard. When you reduce your carb intake and stop consuming foods like pasta and rice for three to four days in a row, your body depletes its glycogen stores substantially. This shifts you into a fat-burning mode. It's important however, to continue fueling your system every 2 to 3 hours to keep your metabolic rate firing. After three to four days, chow a carb-rich meal of pasta or whole grain rice, and you'll shift your body back into a building mode.

Award-winning trainer Billy Beck III, a friend and colleague of mine, utilizes this method with his clients to speed results. He says, "To maximize a client's fat-burning abilities, we often cycle carbohydrates temporarily to deplete glycogen stores, thus forcing the body to rely on stored body fat as an alternative fuel source. It's not uncommon for an individual to experience a 0.5 percent to 1 percent decrease in body fat percentage per week using this type of protocol." Over time and with a little practice, you'll learn to create a sort of "dance" with your body that can result in bigger gains and a leaner physique.

For the recipes in this chapter, I recommend that, to control portion size, you use a smaller bowl than you might normally choose. The fibrous veggies—broccoli, edamame, lima beans, zucchini, yellow squash, onions, tomatoes, asparagus—in these dishes allow you to reduce the amount of pasta you eat while still providing plenty of chow.

ULTIMATE POWER PASTA

The average box of pasta contains 7 grams of protein per serving, and most of us consume at least 2 servings at a time. While 14 grams of protein might sound good, it's incomplete protein. Incomplete proteins are those that lack certain essential amino acids, rendering them useless for muscle building. By adding a small amount of edamame and low-fat cheese, not only do you create a complete (usable) protein, but the soybeans add a little unsaturated fat and fiber to the dish, helping to give the meal a lower glycemic load.

INGREDIENTS:

4	quarts water
1	cup frozen shelled edamame
2	teaspoons extra-virgin olive oil
1	tablespoon dried oregano
1	tablespoon dried basil
1	teaspoon red-pepper flakes
2	cups whole wheat ziti, bow-ties, wheels, or penne
2	cups broccoli florets
2	yellow squash, sliced
2	zucchini, sliced
½	package (3.5 ounces) reduced-fat crumbled feta cheese
4	tablespoons grated Parmesan cheese (optional)

HOW TO MAKE IT:

STEP 1 In a large pot, combine the water, edamame, oil, oregano, basil, and red-pepper flakes. Bring to a boil over high heat.

STEP 2 Add the pasta. Cook for 4 minutes.

STEP 3 Add the broccoli, squash, and zucchini. Cook for 5 to 7 minutes, or until the pasta is al dente.

STEP 4 Drain the pasta and vegetables until dripping but not dry. Add the feta, and toss until completely mixed. Sprinkle on the Parmesan (if using).

Makes 4 servings

Per serving: 347 calories, 18 g protein, 54 g carbohydrates, 8 g total fat, 2 g saturated fat, 9 g fiber, 194 mg sodium

VARIATIONS: You can mix and match just about any vegetables in this dish. Make it colorful with one of the following blends:
- Yellow squash, asparagus, red bell pepper
- Zucchini, mushrooms, yellow squash, no-salt sun-dried tomatoes
- Yellow squash, peas, mushrooms, tomatoes

SIMPLE PASTA 'N' BROCCOLI

You don't have to sacrifice good nutrition for quickness and ease, as this dish proves. It's loaded with high-fiber veggies and flaxseed oil to help control your glycemic response. If I'm trying to lean out, I lower the starchy carbs by making a quick adjustment: Reduce the amount of pasta to 1 heaping cup and add a chopped yellow squash or zucchini to the mix. This way, you'll still keep the volume of food and not feel like you're giving up anything. For an added nutritional benefit, I like to use whole wheat pasta. DeBoles is a brand that you can find just about anywhere.

INGREDIENTS:

4	quarts water
2	teaspoons extra-virgin olive oil
1¾	cup whole wheat rotini or ziti pasta
4	cups broccoli florets
2	tablespoons flaxseed oil
4	teaspoons grated Parmesan cheese

HOW TO MAKE IT:

STEP 1 In a large pot, combine the water and olive oil. Bring to a boil over high heat. Add the pasta. Cook for 5 minutes.

STEP 2 Add the broccoli. Cook for 5 to 7 minutes, or until the pasta is al dente.

STEP 3 Drain. Add the flaxseed oil and toss well.

STEP 4 Divide the pasta among 4 serving bowls. Top each with 1 teaspoon of the cheese.

Makes 4 servings

Per serving: 199 calories, 6 g protein, 22 g carbohydrates, 10.5 g total fat, 1 g saturated fat, 4 g fiber, 49 mg sodium

VARIATION: If you want to kick up the protein a notch, throw in some Ripped Chicken (page 85). Just cut it into strips and toss it in with the finished pasta.

GET CUT WITH CRUCIFERS

Cruciferous vegetables like broccoli, Brussels sprouts, and cabbage contain indole-3-carbinol, a cancer-fighting compound that also helps break down estrogen. For dudes, less estrogen means higher testosterone levels. And that means more muscle!

QUICK ZUCCHINI PASTA

INGREDIENTS:

4	quarts water
2	teaspoons extra-virgin olive oil
1	teaspoon crushed red-pepper flakes
1	teaspoon dried basil
1¾	cups small shell pasta
2	zucchinis, grated
1	cup no-salt tomato sauce
2	tablespoons grated Parmesan cheese
1	teaspoon flaxseed oil

HOW TO MAKE IT:

STEP 1 In a large pot, combine the water, olive oil, red-pepper flakes, and basil. Bring to a boil over high heat.

STEP 2 Add the pasta. Cook for 10 to 12 minutes, or until the pasta is al dente.

STEP 3 In a large bowl, combine the zucchini, tomato sauce, cheese, and flaxseed oil.

STEP 4 Drain the pasta. Add it to the bowl of zucchini sauce. Stir and serve.

Makes 4 servings

Per serving: 231 calories, 8 g protein, 39 g carbohydrates, 5 g total fat, 1 g saturated fat, 3 g fiber, 57 mg sodium

VARIATION: If you want to kick up the protein a notch, add ½ cup frozen edamame to the water and spices.

GET SAUCED

Here are two versions of classic Italian red pasta sauce. The first is the quick and easy sauce that I use nine times out of 10. The second is a high-volume recipe that's great when you're serving a lot of people—well worth the work, with leftovers for days.

EASY SPAGHETTI MEAT SAUCE

1	teaspoon extra-virgin olive oil
½	yellow onion, chopped
1	teaspoon minced garlic
	Pinch of ground black pepper
1	pound extra-lean ground beef
2	cans (8 ounces each) no-salt tomato sauce
¼	teaspoon dried oregano
	Pinch of red-pepper flakes or ground red pepper
	Pinch of dried basil

HOW TO MAKE IT:

STEP 1 Pour the oil into a deep skillet. Swirl the skillet to coat the bottom with oil, then wipe away any excess oil with a paper towel. Heat the skillet over medium-high heat.

STEP 2 Add the onion, garlic, and black pepper. Cook for 1 minute.

STEP 3 Reduce the heat to medium. Add the beef, breaking it apart. Cook over medium-high heat for 6 to 8 minutes, or until the beef is no longer pink.

STEP 4 Add the tomato sauce, oregano, red-pepper flakes, and basil. Bring to a boil, stirring.

STEP 5 Reduce the heat to low. Cook for 5 minutes, stirring occasionally.

Makes 4 servings

Per serving: 193 calories, 24 g protein, 10 g carbohydrates, 6 g total fat, 1.5 g saturated fat, 2 g fiber, 78 mg sodium

CLASSIC SPAGHETTI MEAT SAUCE

2	or 3 cloves garlic, minced
2	large onions, chopped
1	tablespoon extra-virgin olive oil
2	pounds extra-lean ground beef
2	cans (15 ounces each) no-salt tomato puree
2	cans (8 ounces each) no-salt tomato sauce
2	cans (6 ounces each) no-salt tomato paste
3	tablespoons grated Parmesan cheese
1	tablespoon brown sugar
1	tablespoon dried oregano
1	teaspoon ground black pepper

HOW TO MAKE IT:

STEP 1 In a large pot, combine the garlic, onions, and oil. Cook over medium-high heat for 4 to 5 minutes, or until the onions begin to look translucent.

STEP 2 Add the ground beef, breaking it apart. Cook for 6 to 8 minutes, or until no longer pink.

STEP 3 Add the remaining ingredients. Stir. Bring to a boil.

STEP 4 Reduce the heat to low. Cook for 3 hours, stirring occasionally.

Makes 8 servings

Per serving: 258 calories, 27 g protein, 28 g carbohydrates, 5.5 g total fat, 2 g saturated fat, 5 g fiber, 186 mg sodium

PESTO 'N' PASTA

INGREDIENTS:

2	cups ziti
25	leaves fresh basil, finely chopped
2	tablespoons crushed pine nuts
2	tablespoons grated Parmesan cheese
1	tablespoon extra-virgin olive oil
1	tablespoon warm water
1	teaspoon minced garlic

HOW TO MAKE IT:

STEP 1 Cook the pasta according to the package directions.

STEP 2 In a large bowl, mix the remaining ingredients.

STEP 3 Drain the pasta. Pour it into the pesto. Toss until the pasta is coated.

Makes 2 servings

Per serving: 465 calories, 14 g protein, 67 g carbohydrates, 16 g total fat, 2 g saturated fat, 2 g fiber, 85 mg sodium

VARIATIONS:
• Add slices of fresh grilled chicken.
• Add lightly steamed asparagus to the boiling water about 1 minute before the pasta is ready.
• Add fresh cherry tomatoes, halved.

PASTA BOLOGNESE

INGREDIENTS:

4	quarts water
1	teaspoon extra-virgin olive oil
5	dried porcini mushrooms
1	heaping cup rotini, small shells, or ziti
½	pound extra-lean ground beef
1	tablespoon finely chopped yellow onion
1	teaspoon chili powder
1	teaspoon dried basil
	Pinch of ground black pepper
1	can (8 ounces) no-salt tomato sauce
2	tablespoons fat-free ricotta cheese

HOW TO MAKE IT:

STEP 1 In a large pot, combine the water and oil. Bring to a boil over high heat.

STEP 2 Add the mushrooms and pasta. Cook for 10 to 12 minutes, or until the pasta is al dente.

STEP 3 In a nonstick skillet over medium-high heat, combine the ground beef, onion, chili powder, basil, and pepper. Cook, breaking apart the beef, for 6 to 8 minutes, or until the beef is no longer pink. Add the tomato sauce. Bring to a boil. Pour into a large bowl. Add the ricotta and mix.

STEP 4 Drain the pasta and mushrooms. Add to the sauce. Toss.

Makes 2 servings

Per serving: 416 calories, 32 g protein, 52 g carbohydrates, 8 g total fat, 2 g saturated fat, 5 g fiber, 98 mg sodium

SERVING SUGGESTION: For added flavor, top each serving with a little grated Parmesan cheese.

LINGUINE AND LITTLENECKS

This dish has a wonderful aroma from the mix of clams and wine. It makes a nice presentation for a get-together. Sometimes it takes a meal like this to show friends that eating healthy isn't that difficult.

INGREDIENTS:

8	ounces linguine
1	teaspoon extra-virgin olive oil
2	cloves garlic, minced, or 1 tablespoon jarred minced garlic
1	small yellow onion, chopped
	Pinch of red-pepper flakes
1	cup dry white wine
30	littleneck clams, well washed (see note)
1	can (15 ounces) no-salt diced tomatoes
½	cup water, at room temperature (see note)
2	tablespoons chopped dried or fresh parsley

HOW TO MAKE IT:

STEP 1 Cook the pasta according to the package directions. Drain and set aside in a large bowl.

STEP 2 In a large saucepan, add the oil. Heat over medium-high heat. Add the garlic, onion, and red-pepper flakes. Cook for 1 to 2 minutes.

STEP 3 Add the wine. Reduce the heat to medium.

STEP 4 Add the clams, tomatoes, water, and parsley. Stir and cover. Cook for 5 to 6 minutes. The clams will begin to open after about 2 minutes and should take no longer than 6 minutes. Throw away any that haven't opened by that point.

STEP 5 Pour the clam sauce into the bowl with the linguine. Toss to coat.

Makes 4 servings

Per serving: 347 calories, 18 g protein, 51 g carbohydrates, 2.5 g total fat, 0.5 g saturated fat, 3 g fiber, 85 mg sodium

VARIATIONS: Instead of clams, you can also use mussels, which are excellent with this dish. You can also substitute shrimp that have been peeled and deveined. Shrimp will have more flavor if you keep the tails on them. They cook in as little as 1 to 2 minutes, so once they turn white/light pink, they're ready.

NOTE When making the clam sauce, it's important to make sure the water is tepid, because you don't want to interrupt the cooking process by adding cold water. Before cooking clams, discard any that are not tightly shut.

BEEFY LASAGNA

INGREDIENTS:

1	teaspoon extra-virgin olive oil
½	pound extra-lean ground beef
½	small yellow onion, chopped
½	teaspoon dried oregano
	Pinch of ground black pepper
2	cups low-sodium tomato sauce
1	cup fat-free ricotta cheese
1	tablespoon grated Parmesan cheese
6	no-bake lasagna noodles
1	zucchini, thinly sliced

HOW TO MAKE IT:

STEP 1 Preheat the oven to 350°F.

STEP 2 In a nonstick skillet, add the oil. Swirl the skillet to coat the bottom with oil, then wipe away any excess oil with a paper towel. Heat the skillet over medium-high heat.

STEP 3 Add the beef, onion, oregano, and pepper. Cook, breaking apart the beef, for 6 to 8 minutes, or until the beef is no longer pink.

STEP 4 Add the tomato sauce. Bring to a boil. Remove from the heat.

STEP 5 In a bowl, combine the ricotta and Parmesan.

STEP 6 In a 9" × 5" baking dish, layer ½ cup of the sauce, 2 of the noodles, ½ cup of the cheese mix, another ½ cup of the sauce, and ½ of the zucchini. Add another 2 noodles. Repeat the previous layer. Top the zucchini with the remaining ½ cup of sauce.

STEP 7 Cover with foil. Bake for 30 minutes.

STEP 8 Remove the foil. Bake for 15 minutes longer. Remove from the oven and let sit for at least 10 minutes before serving.

Makes 4 servings

Per serving: 324 calories, 24 g protein, 44 g carbohydrates, 4 g total fat, 1 g saturated fat, 4 g fiber, 135 mg sodium

MINI PROTEIN PIES

INGREDIENTS:

2½	cups small shell pasta
¼	teaspoon extra-virgin olive oil
½	small yellow onion, chopped
2	tablespoons chopped red bell pepper
	Pinch of ground black pepper
½	pound extra-lean ground beef
2	medium tomatoes, peeled and chopped
1	can (8 ounces) no-salt tomato sauce
1	teaspoon dried oregano
1	cup fat-free ricotta cheese
¼	cup chopped fresh spinach leaves
1	tablespoon + 1 teaspoon grated Parmesan cheese
¼	cup 4C Carb Careful Plain Breadcrumbs

HOW TO MAKE IT:

STEP 1 Cook the pasta according to the package directions. Drain, rinse, and set aside.

STEP 2 Preheat the oven to 350°F. In a nonstick skillet, add the oil. Swirl the skillet to coat the bottom with oil, then wipe away any excess oil with a paper towel. Heat the skillet over medium-high heat. Add the onion, bell pepper, and black pepper. Cook for 2 minutes.

STEP 3 Add the beef. Cook, breaking apart, for 6 to 8 minutes, or until the beef is no longer pink.

STEP 4 Add the chopped tomatoes, tomato sauce, and oregano. Reduce the heat to low. Cook for 2 to 3 minutes, stirring occasionally.

STEP 5 In a large bowl, combine the ricotta, spinach, and 1 tablespoon Parmesan. Mix well. Add the meat sauce to the bowl and mix.

STEP 6 In each of three personal-size baking dishes (approximately $7\frac{3}{8}$" × $4\frac{7}{8}$" and $1\frac{1}{2}$" to 2" deep), pour a few spoonfuls of the cheesy meat sauce. Evenly divide the pasta shells among the dishes. Top each with an equal amount of the remaining sauce. Bake for 25 minutes.

STEP 7 In a small bowl, mix together the bread crumbs and the remaining 1 teaspoon Parmesan. Raise the oven temperature to broil. Top each protein pie with one-third of the bread crumb mix. Broil for 1 to 2 minutes, or until the crumbs are golden brown.

Makes 3 servings

Per serving: 560 calories, 39 g protein, 77 g carbohydrates, 8 g total fat, 2.5 g saturated fat, 6 g fiber, 209 mg sodium

LEFTOVER TIP: Eat one pie and store the other two in the fridge for up to 3 days. Reheating is easy—just pop it into a toaster oven at 325°F for 15 to 20 minutes.

DISH IT OUT

Personal-size baking dishes can easily be found at your local grocery or department store. They come in a variety of shapes, including oval, square, rectangular, and round. As a personal serving dish that goes from the oven to the table, I think the oval pans make the best presentation, and they come in glass, aluminum, aluminum foil, nonstick, ceramic, and stone. Aluminum foil pans are disposable, so there's little to no cleanup, but the other types will last forever, saving you money in the long run. Look for dishes that are about $1\frac{1}{2}$" to 2" deep, with widths of around $7\frac{3}{8}$" × $4\frac{7}{8}$", 8" × 4", or 9" × 5".

EGGPLANT LASAGNA

INGREDIENTS:

1	cup fat-free ricotta cheese
1	tablespoon grated Parmesan cheese
2	cups low-sodium tomato sauce
½	can (2.25 ounces) sliced black olives, drained
1	eggplant, peeled and sliced into ¼"-thick rounds
6	no-bake lasagna noodles
1	small tomato, sliced into ¼"-thick rounds
½	red bell pepper, sliced into very thin rounds

HOW TO MAKE IT:

STEP 1 Preheat the oven to 350°F.

STEP 2 In a small bowl, mix together the ricotta and Parmesan.

STEP 3 In a medium bowl, mix together the tomato sauce and olives.

STEP 4 In a 9" × 5" baking dish, layer ¼ cup of the tomato sauce, 2 of the eggplant rounds, 2 of the noodles, ⅓ cup of the cheese mix, one-quarter of the tomatoes, and one-third of the peppers. Repeat the layers two times. Top with the remaining ¼ cup sauce and one-quarter tomatoes.

STEP 5 Cover with foil. Bake for 30 minutes.

STEP 6 Remove the foil. Bake for 15 minutes longer. Remove from the oven and let sit for at least 10 minutes before serving.

Makes 4 servings

Per serving: 247 calories, 10 g protein, 48 g carbohydrates, 3 g total fat, 1 g saturated fat, 8 g fiber, 119 mg sodium

PASTA SALAD

INGREDIENTS:

1	box (16 ounces) bow-tie pasta
1	can (8 ounces) chickpeas, drained and rinsed
1	can (2.25 ounces) sliced black olives, drained
2	ribs celery, chopped
2	cucumbers, peeled, seeded, and cut into chunks
½	cup shredded carrots
⅓	cup chopped sweet onion
2	tablespoons shredded Parmesan cheese
3	tablespoons extra-virgin olive oil
½	cup red wine vinegar
½	teaspoon Worcestershire sauce
½	teaspoon spicy brown mustard
½	heaping teaspoon jarred minced garlic
2	tablespoons chopped fresh Italian parsley
1	tablespoon chopped fresh basil or 1 teaspoon dried
¼	teaspoon ground black pepper

HOW TO MAKE IT:

STEP 1 Cook the pasta according to the package directions. Drain. Rinse under cool water for 30 seconds, then put in a large bowl.

STEP 2 Add the remaining ingredients and mix well.

STEP 3 Cover and refrigerate overnight (or for at least 4 hours). Mix before serving.

Makes 15 servings

Per serving: 165 calories, 5 g protein, 28 g carbohydrates, 4 g total fat, 1 g saturated fat, 2 g fiber, 91 mg sodium

TIP Rinsing pasta with cool water removes excess starch and keeps the pasta from sticking together. It also quickly cools the pasta to stop further cooking—and that speeds up the recipe preparation.

BASIC COUSCOUS SALAD

INGREDIENTS:

1	box (12 ounces) couscous
	Juice of 2 lemons
½	teaspoon lemon zest
2	tablespoons honey
1	tablespoon Dijon mustard
1	teaspoon extra-virgin olive oil
1	container (3.5 ounces) crumbled low-fat feta cheese
3	plum tomatoes, chopped
1	medium cucumber, seeded and cut into chunks
½	onion, finely chopped
1	can (2.25 ounces) sliced black olives, drained and rinsed
¼	teaspoon ground black pepper
½	cup coarsely chopped dried or fresh parsley
8	leaves Bibb lettuce

HOW TO MAKE IT:

STEP 1 Cook the couscous according to the package directions.

STEP 2 In a small bowl, combine the lemon juice, lemon zest, honey, mustard, and oil. Mix well.

STEP 3 In a large bowl, combine the couscous, cheese, tomatoes, cucumber, onion, olives, pepper, and parsley. Add the lemon-honey sauce and mix.

STEP 4 Place the lettuce leaves on 8 salad plates. Top each with equal portions of the couscous salad. Serve at room temperature or chilled.

Makes 8 servings

Per serving: 233 calories, 9 g protein, 43 g carbohydrates, 3.5 g total fat, 1 g saturated fat, 3 g fiber, 287 mg sodium

SERVING SUGGESTION: This makes a nice side dish to any fish, chicken, or beef meal. It keeps in the fridge for up to a week—if you don't eat it before then.

ADD A LITTLE ZEST TO YOUR LIFE

Lemon zest is just grated lemon rind. The best way to achieve a nice zest is to buy a specific tool called—drumroll, please—a zester. You can easily find one at any grocery store, large department store, or cooking supply shop.

VEGETABLE-PACKED ISRAELI COUSCOUS

I like using the larger, pearl-size Israeli couscous because it's so versatile. You can mix in many combinations of veggies, herbs, and even fruits, and it comes out great every time. Couscous is made from semolina, and therefore it's considered a pasta. You cook it just like other pastas.

INGREDIENTS:

2	cups Israeli couscous
10	grape or cherry tomatoes, halved
½	yellow bell pepper, seeded and chopped
1	cup shelled edamame
⅓	cup dried cranberries
¼	cup chopped dried or fresh parsley
	Juice of 2 lemons
1	teaspoon extra-virgin olive oil
	Ground black pepper to taste

HOW TO MAKE IT:

STEP 1 Cook the couscous according to the package directions. Drain. Rinse well under cold running water. Place in a large bowl.

STEP 2 Add the remaining ingredients and mix well. Serve either at room temperature or chilled.

Makes 6 servings

Per serving: 157 calories, 7 g protein, 24 g carbohydrates, 2 g total fat, 0 g saturated fat, 5 g fiber, 56 mg sodium

SERVING SUGGESTION: This dish can be eaten as a meal, a snack, or an accompaniment to any protein-based meal.

VARIATION: For a change of pace, you can replace the edamame, tomatoes, and/or yellow bell pepper with any three of the following: ½ red bell pepper, seeded and chopped; ½ orange bell pepper, seeded and chopped; ½ onion, chopped; 1 cucumber, seeded and cut into chunks; 1 cup chopped baby carrots; 1 rib celery, chopped; or 15 asparagus spears, trimmed, chopped, and lightly steamed.

The dried cranberries can be swapped out for ⅓ cup raisins, golden raisins, or chopped dried apricots.

THE FASTEST RICE AND VEGGIE DISH EVER

You get home from a long day at work, your stomach is empty, your blood sugar is low, and you're just not in a good mood. You might be tempted to grab an overprocessed snack or some other kind of empty carbohydrate to soothe those feelings. Carbohydrates are not only energy for your body, they're also the primary source of fuel for your brain. That's why eating a high-carbohydrate food will help your mood and allow you to think more clearly.

At times like this, function is more important than form. You need an easy meal that satisfies your need for carbs but balances them with lean protein to keep the glycemic load low. This complete meal takes only 15 minutes from start to your first mouthful. And since you cook everything in one pot, there's hardly any cleanup.

INGREDIENTS:

2½	cups water	1	medium zucchini, chopped
1	teaspoon extra-virgin olive oil	1	medium yellow squash, chopped
½	teaspoon McCormick Imitation Butter Flavor		Pinch of no-salt lemon-pepper seasoning
1	cup basmati or jasmine rice		1 can (4 ounces) low-sodium chunk white tuna packed in water, drained and rinsed, or 1 package (14 ounces) low-fat firm tofu, drained and crumbled (see notes)
2	stalks broccoli, chopped	1	tablespoon grated Parmesan cheese

HOW TO WORK WITH TOFU

Sometimes tofu needs a little help—particularly when it's not mixed into a soup or other liquid dish and you want it to be dry and firm. Here's how to handle it.

- Split a block of extra-firm tofu in half by carefully cutting it down the middle from end-to-end.
- Wrap each half in several paper towels and lightly press to draw water from the tofu.
- Store in the fridge (still wrapped in the towels) for 15 to 30 minutes with something stacked on top (a heavy skillet or a gallon of milk will do just fine), to press out as much moisture as possible.
- When fully dehydrated, this pressed tofu will be perfect for grilling or baking.

HOW TO MAKE IT:

STEP 1 In a medium saucepan over high heat, combine the water, oil, and butter flavor. Bring to a boil.

STEP 2 Add the rice and stir. Return to a boil.

STEP 3 Add the broccoli, zucchini, squash, and lemon-pepper seasoning. Return to a boil. Stir.

STEP 4 Cover. Reduce the heat to low. Cook for 10 to 15 minutes, or until all the water has been absorbed.

STEP 5 Fluff with a fork. Pour into a large bowl. Add the tuna or tofu. Mix. Top with the cheese.

Makes 3 servings

Per serving with **tuna**: 354 calories, 17 g protein, 69 g carbohydrates, 3.5 g total fat, 1 g saturated fat, 6 g fiber, 86 mg sodium

Per serving with **tofu**: 330 calories, 14 g protein, 70 g carbohydrates, 3 g total fat, 1 g saturated fat, 6 g fiber, 91 mg sodium

VARIATIONS: Other veggie options include shelled edamame, peas, green beans, spinach, mushrooms, low-sodium sun-dried tomatoes, asparagus, or any other vegetable you can think of. Experiment and have fun with it.

NOTE You can eat the tuna separately from the rice and veggies, or finely break it apart in the bowl by using a fork. I often drizzle a little balsamic vinegar directly into the can to boost the flavor, and then I eat the tuna while the rice and veggies are cooking.

If you use flavored tofu, be sure to read the label and choose a lower-sodium flavor.

BAKED CREAMY RICE

This dish calls for Arborio rice, which cooks up creamier than other kinds of rice because it has more starch. Look for it in the Italian foods aisle of your supermarket.

INGREDIENTS:

1	**cup Arborio rice**
1	**can (15 ounces) no-salt black soybeans, rinsed and drained (see note)**
1	**can (14.5 ounces) low-sodium chicken broth**
⅓	**cup dried porcini mushrooms (about 15 pieces)**
¼	**cup chopped onion**
1	**package (14 ounces) low-fat soft silken tofu, drained**
¼	**cup pine nuts**
1	**tablespoon dried or fresh parsley**

HOW TO MAKE IT:

STEP 1 Preheat the oven to 350°F. In a 2½-quart baking dish, combine the rice, soybeans, broth, mushrooms, and onion.

STEP 2 In a bowl, whisk the tofu until smooth. Add to the rice mixture. Cover with foil. Bake for 45 minutes.

STEP 3 In a skillet coated with cooking spray, toast the pine nuts over medium heat until lightly browned. Or, put the pine nuts on aluminum foil and broil in a toaster oven for 1 minute, or until lightly browned. Watch them because they are oily and will toast very quickly. Set aside.

STEP 4 When the rice mixture is ready, remove from the oven and stir well to fully mix in the tofu. This will make the dish even creamier. Fold in the toasted pine nuts and parsley.

Makes 6 servings

Per serving: 275 calories, 16 g protein, 36 g carbohydrates, 9 g total fat, 1 g saturated fat, 6 g fiber, 71 mg sodium

NOTE I like Eden Organic Black Soy Beans because, as the name says, they're organic, they consistently taste fresh, and they contain little to no sodium per serving.

TABBOULEH SALAD

INGREDIENTS:

1½	**cups boiling water**
1	**cup bulgur wheat**
½	**yellow onion, chopped**
¼	**green bell pepper, chopped**
1	**tablespoon extra-virgin olive oil**
¼	**teaspoon ground black pepper**
2	**bunches fresh parsley, finely chopped**
2	**tomatoes, seeded and chopped**
1	**cucumber, peeled and chopped**
	Juice of 2 lemons
½	**can (2.25 ounces) sliced black olives, drained**

HOW TO MAKE IT:

STEP 1 In a large bowl, combine the water and bulgur. Stir. Cover and let sit for 30 minutes, or until the bulgur has soaked up the water.

STEP 2 Add the onion, bell pepper, oil, and black pepper. Toss. Refrigerate for 1 hour.

STEP 3 Add the parsley, tomatoes, cucumber, lemon juice, and olives. Toss.

Makes 6 servings

Per serving: 137 calories, 4 g protein, 24 g carbohydrates, 4 g total fat, 0.5 g saturated fat, 6 g fiber, 97 mg sodium

TOFU BULGUR SALAD

INGREDIENTS:

1½	cups boiling water
1	cup bulgur wheat
2	plum tomatoes, seeded and chopped
1	bunch fresh parsley, coarsely chopped
	Juice of 1–2 lemons
½	cup no-salt chickpeas, rinsed and drained
3	teaspoons extra-virgin olive oil
½	yellow onion, chopped
¼	cup chopped yellow bell pepper
1	package (14 ounces) low-fat extra-firm tofu, drained and cubed
¼	teaspoon no-salt lemon-pepper seasoning
1	avocado, cubed

HOW TO MAKE IT:

STEP 1 In a large bowl, combine the water and bulgur. Stir. Cover and let sit for 30 minutes, or until the bulgur has soaked up the water.

STEP 2 Add the tomatoes, parsley, lemon juice, chickpeas, 2 teaspoons of the oil, half of the onion, and half of the bell pepper. Toss well.

STEP 3 In a nonstick skillet, add the remaining 1 teaspoon olive oil. Swirl the skillet to coat the bottom with oil, then wipe away any excess oil with a paper towel. Heat the skillet over medium-high heat. Add the tofu, lemon-pepper seasoning, the remaining onion, and the remaining bell pepper. Cook for 5 to 8 minutes, or until the tofu is browned.

STEP 4 Add the tofu mixture and the avocado to the bulgur mixture. Gently fold together.

STEP 5 Refrigerate for at least 3 hours. Gently toss before serving.

Makes 6 servings

Per serving: 219 calories, 10 g protein, 28 g carbohydrates, 8.5 g total fat, 1 g saturated fat, 8 g fiber, 77 mg sodium

PROTEIN-RICH QUINOA SALAD

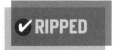

More and more people are learning about exotic grains like quinoa, amaranth, and buckwheat—and for good reason. Quinoa (pronounced keen-wa) is a nice source of protein, yielding the highest amount (18 grams per cup) of any grain. It's also a complete protein, containing all eight essential amino acids, which is uncommon for a grain and usually true only of animal proteins like beef, poultry, fish, eggs, and dairy. When cooked, quinoa will open and reveal its spiral-shaped germ ring. This ring is the gold nugget because that's where the majority of the protein lies. It also contains an array of other nutrients, including potassium to help the body's water balance, B vitamins for energy production, magnesium and lysine for better calcium and potassium absorption, zinc for hormone production, and fiber to help shuttle fats out of your system. The best part is that it really doesn't take that long to prepare—about 15 minutes.

INGREDIENTS:

1	cup quinoa (see note)
2	plum tomatoes, chopped
1	bunch fresh parsley, coarsely chopped
½	cucumber, seeded and chopped
¼	cup finely chopped red onion
1	tablespoon extra-virgin olive oil
	Juice of 2 key limes (or ½ lemon or lime)
	Ground black pepper to taste

HOW TO MAKE IT:

STEP 1 Cook the quinoa according to the package directions. Let it cool in a large bowl for about 30 minutes.

STEP 2 Add the remaining ingredients. Mix. Eat cold or at room temperature.

Makes 6 servings

Per serving: 140 calories, 4 g protein, 22 g carbohydrates, 4 g total fat, 0.5 g saturated fat, 2 g fiber, 10 mg sodium

RIPPED TIP

If you're going to prepare this recipe in a Ripped Phase, limit it to one time throughout the two-week period.

NOTE

Before you cook quinoa, always rinse it until the water runs clear, to get rid of its natural bitter coating.

10

SOUP, VEGGIES & SALADS

Muscle Chow is all about eating a well-balanced diet full of quality proteins, whole grains, and healthy fats in order to set the best possible stage for optimum muscle growth. So while animal proteins are an important foundation, foods from plant sources are the supporting cast that help achieve nutritional balance. Vegetables and fruits provide fiber and antioxidants to help with digestion and to keep your disease-fighting system in peak form.

The following side dishes will help add texture and color to enhance the taste and presentation of any protein-rich meal. For instance, prepare the Beefcake Meat Loaf (page 61) and pair it with the Pear-Walnut Salad (page 176). Or pick any of the side dishes, like the Classic Steamed Veggies (page 154) or Baked Asparagus with Sea Salt (page 161), to go with the Simple Baked Lemon-Pepper Chicken (page 75). For the perfect complement to any of the grilled seafood dishes in Chapter 8, try the Veggie Kebabs (page 158). You'll find that I offer serving suggestions for many of the main-dish recipes, but I encourage you to be creative, mix and match with these sides, and discover food combinations that will become your favorites for years to come.

LOADED SOUP

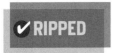

This recipe is super easy, and that's only half of what makes it so good. Loaded Soup is also a solid recovery snack because it has phytochemicals from the organic veggies and protein from the tofu. Phytochemicals are antioxidants in vegetables and fruits that are powerful cancer fighters, support the immune system, and help reduce inflammation. Because soybeans are one of the very few legumes that contain all the essential amino acids, soybean-based tofu is a nice source of complete protein. Soy is also an excellent source of L-glutamine, a nutrient that helps with muscle recovery and repair. It contains almost twice as much L-glutamine per serving as whey protein does.

INGREDIENTS:

1   can (15 ounces) Health Valley No Salt Added Organic Mushroom Barley Soup

1   cup firm or extra-firm light tofu, drained and cubed

1   teaspoon ground black pepper

HOW TO MAKE IT:

STEP 1 In a large saucepan, combine the soup and tofu. Bring to a boil over medium-high heat, stirring occasionally.

STEP 2 Add the pepper. Reduce the heat to low. Cook for 3 to 5 minutes.

Makes 1 serving

Per serving: 210 calories, 11 g protein, 33 g carbohydrates, 4.5 g total fat, 0 g saturated fat, 6 g fiber, 220 mg sodium

VARIATION: Loaded Soup is just as good when made with one of the other types of Health Valley no-salt-added organic soups. Some of the other varieties worth trying are vegetable, minestrone, potato leek, lentil, and split pea. Health Valley also offers no-salt-added chilis, including spicy vegetarian and mild vegetarian. All of these products are made with all-natural ingredients that are certified USDA organic. None of them contain artificial colors, flavors, or preservatives, and you won't find hydrogenated oils, partially hydrogenated oils, or trans fats in any of the Health Valley products.

CLASSIC STEAMED VEGGIES

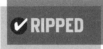 **RIPPED**

INGREDIENTS:

2	**cups broccoli florets**
1	**medium zucchini, sliced**
1	**medium yellow squash, sliced**
½	**teaspoon extra-virgin olive oil**
	No-salt lemon-pepper seasoning

HOW TO MAKE IT:

STEP 1 Place a steamer basket in a large pot with 2" of water. Bring to a boil over high heat. Place the broccoli, zucchini, and squash in the basket.

STEP 2 Drizzle the oil over the veggies. Sprinkle the lemon-pepper seasoning (to taste) over the top.

STEP 3 Steam for 5 minutes, or until the veggies are slightly tender.

Makes 2 servings

Per serving: 66 calories, 4 g protein, 11 g carbohydrates, 1.5 g total fat, 0 g saturated fat, 5 g fiber, 43 mg sodium

FRIENDLY FIBER

The recommended daily intake of fiber is about 30 grams, so I try to get at least that amount (or more) each day. Fiber helps clear your body of toxins by moving bulk through the intestines, helps control cholesterol levels, and shuttles excess fat from your system. It also helps regulate blood sugar by slowing down digestion, plus it helps make you feel full so you don't overeat. Sources include fresh vegetables and fruits (especially when the skin is left on), whole grains, legumes, nuts, and seeds. While most of these foods are carbohydrate-based, their fiber content makes them slow-digesting carbs. Their slow absorption rate creates a sort of timed-release effect that helps control your body's insulin response.

FASTER THAN A STEAM LOCOMOTIVE

Ripped Phase

For a super-quick side dish, it's easy to steam fresh vegetables in the microwave. Here's how I prepare a few of my favorites.

Broccoli: Put 2 to 3 cups broccoli florets in a microwaveable bowl, top them off with a sprinkle of no-salt lemon-pepper seasoning , and add ¼ cup water. Cover with plastic wrap. Pierce six small holes to vent. Microwave on high power for 3½ to 4 minutes, or until tender. Drain off the excess water, then top with fat-free pump-spray butter.

Green beans: Put 2 cups fresh-cut green beans in a microwaveable bowl, top them off with a sprinkle of no-salt lemon-pepper seasoning, and add ¼ cup water. Cover with plastic wrap. Pierce six small holes to vent. Microwave on high power for 4½ to 5 minutes, or until crisp-tender. Drain off the excess water, then top with fat-free pump-spray butter or 1 teaspoon flaxseed oil. Toss to coat.

Cauliflower: Put 2 to 3 cups cauliflower florets in a microwaveable bowl, top them off with a pinch of ground black pepper, and add ¼ cup water. Cover with plastic wrap. Pierce six small holes to vent. Microwave on high power for 3½ to 4 minutes, or until tender. Drain off the excess water, then top with fat-free pump-spray butter.

Corn on the cob: Remove the husk and silk from an ear of corn. Wash the ear and, without drying, wrap it in a paper towel. Place it on a microwaveable plate. Microwave on high power for 4 minutes. To steam 2 ears of corn, wrap each separately and microwave for 3 minutes, then turn both ears and microwave for 3 minutes longer, or until the kernels are tender. Top with some fat-free pump-spray butter and a little ground black pepper.

GREEN PROTEIN

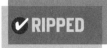 **RIPPED**

INGREDIENTS:

1   cup frozen shelled edamame

1   cup frozen lima beans

1   teaspoon extra-virgin olive oil

         Pinch of ground black pepper

2–4   cups fresh broccoli florets

HOW TO MAKE IT:

STEP 1 Fill a pot with 2" of water. Add the edamame, lima beans, oil, and pepper. Bring to a boil over high heat.

STEP 2 Add the broccoli and stir. Cover and boil for 1 minute.

STEP 3 Remove from the heat. Let sit, covered, for 3 minutes. Drain.

Makes 2 servings

Per serving: 215 calories, 16 g protein, 30 g carbohydrates, 4 g total fat, 0.5 g saturated fat, 11 g fiber, 75 mg sodium

SERVING SUGGESTION: Boost the flavor by squeezing a lemon wedge or sprinkling a little grated Parmesan cheese over top.

TIP In order to keep the sodium low in this dish, be sure to read labels and choose lima bean and edamame brands that have the lowest sodium per serving.

HONEY-ROASTED VEGGIE MIX

INGREDIENTS:

½ red bell pepper, cut into 1" pieces

1 teaspoon extra-virgin olive oil

¼ teaspoon dried thyme

Pinch of sea salt

¼ teaspoon + 1 pinch of ground black pepper

10 cherry tomatoes, halved

1 medium zucchini, cut into chunks

1 medium yellow squash, cut into chunks

2 tablespoons honey

½ pound asparagus spears, with bottoms cut off

1 cup frozen shelled edamame

HOW TO MAKE IT:

STEP 1 Preheat the oven to 450°F. Place the bell pepper in a 12" × 9" baking pan. Add the oil and toss to coat.

STEP 2 Sprinkle with the thyme, salt, and ¼ teaspoon black pepper. Toss to coat.

STEP 3 Roast for 5 minutes.

STEP 4 Add the tomatoes, zucchini, squash, and honey. Toss to mix.

STEP 5 Roast for 5 minutes.

STEP 6 Add the asparagus and toss.

STEP 7 Roast for 10 to 15 minutes, or until all the veggies are tender.

STEP 8 While the other veggies are roasting, add the edamame and the pinch of black pepper to a small saucepan filled halfway with water. Boil over medium-high heat for 5 minutes, or until tender.

STEP 9 Drain the edamame and place in a large bowl. Add the roasted vegetables to the bowl and toss.

Makes 6 servings

Per serving: 90 calories, 5 g protein, 15 g carbohydrates, 2 g total fat, 0 g saturated fat, 4 g fiber, 45 mg sodium

VEGGIE KEBABS

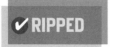 **RIPPED**

Some people soak kebabs in a high-sodium bottled marinade before grilling them. Since you're eating Muscle Chow, you're not one of those guys. This recipe leaves out the excess sodium. You'll lightly brush the kebabs with some olive oil, then spark their natural flavors with ground black pepper and no-salt lemon-pepper seasoning.

INGREDIENTS:

2	**zucchini, cut into chunks**
2	**yellow squash, cut into chunks**
1	**orange bell pepper, cut into 1" squares**
1	**sweet onion, cut into 1" squares**
1	**pint grape or cherry tomatoes**
1	**pint small mushrooms (about 20)**
4	**tablespoons extra-virgin olive oil**
	Ground black pepper
	No-salt lemon-pepper seasoning

RIPPED TIP

If you're preparing this recipe in a Ripped Phase, substitute olive oil spray for the olive oil.

HOW TO MAKE IT:

STEP 1 Soak 20 wooden skewers in water for 30 minutes. This will keep the skewers from burning on the grill. Preheat the grill to medium-low.

STEP 2 Evenly divide the zucchini, squash, bell pepper, onion, tomatoes, and mushrooms among the skewers.

STEP 3 Lightly brush each kebab with the oil. Lightly season with the black pepper and lemon-pepper seasoning (to taste).

STEP 4 Grill for 10 to 12 minutes, rotating every 3 to 4 minutes, or until slightly charred and tender.

Makes 4 servings

Per serving: 190 calories, 5 g protein, 15 g carbohydrates, 14 g total fat, 2 g saturated fat, 4 g fiber, 25 mg sodium

TIP I like to use wooden skewers instead of metal simply because veggies tend to rotate less while you're turning them on the grill. Also, wooden skewers are cheap, so you can toss them when you're done.

VEGGIE PANCAKES

This is quick and easy to do and makes a great protein meal any time of the day.

INGREDIENTS:

6	egg whites
½	cup unsalted matzo meal
2	medium zucchini, grated
½	yellow onion, grated
1	teaspoon chopped dried or fresh parsley
	Pinch of ground black pepper
½	teaspoon minced garlic
1	teaspoon extra-virgin olive oil

HOW TO MAKE IT:

STEP 1 In a large bowl, combine the egg whites and matzo meal. Mix.

STEP 2 In another large bowl, combine the zucchini, onion, parsley, pepper, and garlic. Add the egg mixture and stir until well mixed.

STEP 3 In a large skillet, add the oil. Swirl the skillet to coat the bottom with oil. Lightly wipe away the excess with a paper towel and set aside the towel. Use this towel to wipe the skillet between pancakes, recoating the skillet with the oil and cleaning away any pancake batter crumbs.

STEP 4 Preheat the skillet to medium. To determine whether the skillet is the right temperature, flick in a drop of water. If the drop bounces when it hits the skillet, the skillet is ready. If it bounces out of the skillet, the skillet is too hot.

STEP 5 Add a spoonful of the batter to the skillet, spreading it with the back of the spoon to create a 6" pancake. Cook for 3 minutes. Flip. Cook for 3 minutes longer.

STEP 6 Repeat Step 5 with the remaining batter to make a total of 6 pancakes.

Makes 6 pancakes

Per pancake: 80 calories, 6 g protein, 12 g carbohydrates, 1 g total fat, 0 g saturated fat, 1 g fiber, 62 mg sodium

TIP To keep the pancakes warm while you cook the rest of the batter, place them on a baking sheet or sheet of aluminum foil in a 175°F oven.

FRESH GREEN BEANS WITH ALMONDS

INGREDIENTS:

1	pound fresh green beans, washed and trimmed
½	teaspoon extra-virgin olive oil
	Pinch of sea salt
	Pinch of ground black pepper
⅓	cup slivered almonds

HOW TO MAKE IT:

STEP 1 Bring a large pot of water to a boil over high heat. Add the green beans. Boil for 2 to 4 minutes, or until crisp-tender. Drain.

STEP 2 Place the beans in a large bowl. Add the oil, salt, and pepper. Toss to coat.

STEP 3 In a large nonstick skillet, coat the almonds with butter-flavored cooking spray. Heat over medium-high heat for 2 to 3 minutes, stirring frequently, or until browned.

STEP 4 Reduce the heat to medium. Add the beans. Cook for 2 minutes, stirring.

Makes 4 servings

Per serving: 85 calories, 3 g protein, 9 g carbohydrates, 5 g total fat, 0.5 g saturated fat, 5 g fiber, 37 mg sodium

BAKED ASPARAGUS WITH SEA SALT

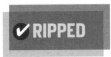 **RIPPED**

INGREDIENTS:

1   **bunch fresh asparagus spears, with bottoms cut off**

1   **teaspoon extra-virgin olive oil**

    Pinch of sea salt

HOW TO MAKE IT:

STEP 1 Place the asparagus in a 12" × 9" baking dish. Add the oil and toss to coat. Sprinkle with the salt and toss.

STEP 2 Put into the oven. Turn on the broiler and broil for 2 minutes. Shake the dish to turn the asparagus. Cook for asparagus 1 to 2 minutes longer, or until slightly browned.

Makes 4 servings

Per serving: 24 calories, 1 g protein, 3 g carbohydrates, 1 g total fat, 0 g saturated fat, 1 g fiber, 40 mg sodium

RIPPED TIP

If you're preparing this recipe in a Ripped Phase, substitute no-salt lemon pepper for the sea salt. It's also important to note that asparagus is a good diuretic, which can help rid the water between your skin and muscle to allow for a more ripped look.

OVEN-ROASTED ZUCCHINI

INGREDIENTS:

4   **medium zucchini, quarter-cut lengthwise, then cut in half widthwise**

1   **teaspoon extra-virgin olive oil**

1   **teaspoon no-salt lemon-pepper seasoning**

HOW TO MAKE IT:

STEP 1 Preheat the oven to 450°F. Place the zucchini in a large baking dish. Add the oil and toss to coat.

STEP 2 Add the lemon-pepper seasoning and toss.

STEP 3 Bake for 10 minutes. Toss.

STEP 4 Bake for 10 minutes longer, or until tender.

STEP 5 Raise the oven temperature to broil. Broil for 3 to 5 minutes, or until browned but not burned.

Makes 4 servings

Per serving: 43 calories, 2 g protein, 7 g carbohydrates, 1.5 g total fat, 0 g saturated fat, 2 g fiber, 29 mg sodium

VARIATION: Use yellow squash or equal portions of yellow squash and zucchini.

RIPPED TIP

If you're preparing this recipe in a Ripped Phase, substitute olive oil spray for the olive oil.

BAKED YELLOW SQUASH

INGREDIENTS:

1	teaspoon extra-virgin olive oil
2	egg whites
½	cup fat-free milk
⅔	cup 4C Carb Careful Plain Breadcrumbs
1	tablespoon shredded Parmesan cheese
½	teaspoon dried minced onion
½	teaspoon paprika
½	teaspoon dried or fresh parsley
¼	teaspoon garlic powder
¼	teaspoon ground black pepper
2	large yellow squash, quarter-cut lengthwise, then cut in half widthwise

HOW TO MAKE IT:

STEP 1 Preheat the oven to 450°F. Pour the oil into a large baking dish. Swirl to coat the bottom of the dish. Wipe away any excess with a paper towel.

STEP 2 In a shallow dish, mix together the egg whites and milk.

STEP 3 In another shallow dish, combine the bread crumbs, cheese, onion, paprika, parsley, garlic powder, and pepper. Stir well to mix.

STEP 4 Dredge the squash in the egg mixture and then in the crumb mixture. Place in the baking dish cut side up.

STEP 5 Bake for 15 minutes, or until browned.

Makes 4 servings

Per serving: 118 calories, 14 g protein, 12 g carbohydrates, 2 g total fat, 0.5 g saturated fat, 4 g fiber, 68 mg sodium

ROASTED ACORN SQUASH

INGREDIENTS:

2	small acorn squash, cut in half lengthwise and seeded
1	apple, chopped
4	teaspoons brown sugar
4	teaspoons water
1	teaspoon extra-virgin olive oil
⅛	teaspoon ground cinnamon
	Ground black pepper

HOW TO MAKE IT:

STEP 1 Preheat the oven to 400°F. Place the squash cut side down in a large baking dish. Add ¼" of water.

STEP 2 Roast for 35 minutes.

STEP 3 In a small bowl, mix together the apple, brown sugar, water, oil, and cinnamon.

STEP 4 Divide the apple mixture evenly between the squash halves. Sprinkle each half with a pinch of pepper.

STEP 5 Roast for 20 minutes, or until fork-tender.

STEP 6 Raise the oven temperature to broil. Broil for 2 to 3 minutes, or until lightly browned.

Makes 4 servings

Per serving: 132 calories, 2 g protein, 32 g carbohydrates, 1.5 g total fat, 0 g saturated fat, 4 g fiber, 9 mg sodium

BAKED CAULIFLOWER

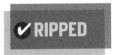
✔ RIPPED

INGREDIENTS:

1	**head cauliflower, chopped**
1	**teaspoon extra-virgin olive oil**
1	**teaspoon dried or fresh parsley**
¼	**teaspoon ground black pepper**
1	**tablespoon grated Parmesan cheese**

HOW TO MAKE IT:

STEP 1 Preheat the oven to 450°F. Place the cauliflower in a large baking dish. Add the oil and toss to coat.

STEP 2 Bake for 10 minutes. Stir, then bake for 10 minutes longer.

STEP 3 Sprinkle with the parsley and pepper. Bake for 5 minutes, or until slightly browned.

STEP 4 Sprinkle with the cheese. Mix well.

Makes 4 servings

Per serving: 52 calories, 3 g protein, 8 g carbohydrates, 1.5 g total fat, 0.5 g saturated fat, 4 g fiber, 62 mg sodium

RIPPED TIP

If you want to prepare this recipe in a Ripped Phase, substitute olive oil spray for the olive oil and omit the Parmesan cheese.

ROASTED HEIRLOOM CARROTS

Whenever I find these carrots, grown from vintage seeds rather than by large agribusiness farms, they're hard to pass up without buying a bundle or three. Often called heirloom or rainbow carrots, they're most readily available at farmers' markets and health food stores that sell a wide variety of vegetables. They look like the ones Bugs Bunny walked around with because they still have the stems attached and they're usually smaller than conventional carrots. They come in a variety of colors besides orange, including red, yellow, and even purple, indicating that they're high in lycopene and beta-carotene—antioxidants that offer health benefits such as immune support, growth and repair of tissues, and hormone balance.

INGREDIENTS:

2	pounds heirloom carrots, trimmed of all but ½" stem
1	teaspoon extra-virgin olive oil
	Pinch of sea salt
½	teaspoon ground black pepper
	Pinch of thyme
2	ounces fresh goat cheese, chopped (optional)

HOW TO MAKE IT:

STEP 1 Preheat the oven to 450°F. Place the carrots in a 12" × 9" baking dish. Add the oil and toss to coat.

STEP 2 Sprinkle with the salt, pepper, and thyme. Toss.

STEP 3 Roast for 25 minutes, turning every 8 minutes, or until brown on all sides and tender.

STEP 4 Sprinkle with the cheese, if using.

Makes 6 servings

Per serving: 70 calories, 1 g protein, 15 g carbohydrates, 1 g total fat, 0 g saturated fat, 4 g fiber, 129 mg sodium

VARIATION: For a little extra color and flavor, add cherry or grape tomatoes during the final 5 to 8 minutes of roasting.

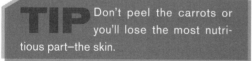

TIP Don't peel the carrots or you'll lose the most nutritious part—the skin.

SUPERHERO SWEETS

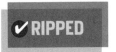
✔ RIPPED

Sweet potatoes are the best example of Muscle Chow's approach to carbs. They're loaded with complex carbohydrates to help replenish glycogen stores after a hard training session. They're also packed with antioxidants like beta-carotene, vitamin C, and potassium to help your immune system, and they're a good source of dietary fiber (especially if you eat the skin). This makes Superhero Sweets a low-glycemic dish that provides sustained fuel to help you feel more energized over long periods of time. These Superhero Sweets are super easy, super basic, and super good!

INGREDIENTS:

3   or 4 medium sweet potatoes

½   teaspoon extra-virgin olive oil

HOW TO MAKE IT:

STEP 1 Preheat the oven to 450°F. Rub each potato with a small amount of the oil. Make a 3" cut through the skin of each potato.

STEP 2 Place in a baking pan. Bake for 1 hour, or until a fork inserted easily goes to the middle.

Makes 4 servings

Per serving: 145 calories, 2 g protein, 32 g carbohydrates, 0.5 g total fat, 0 g saturated fat, 4 g fiber, 45 mg sodium

RIPPED TIP

If you're preparing this recipe in a Ripped Phase, you may choose to substitute olive oil spray for the olive oil.

TIP The potatoes will keep for up to 4 days when cooled, wrapped in plastic wrap, and refrigerated. I like to top them with a little fat-free pump-spray butter and chow them cold or reheated in the microwave for a minute or two. They make a great postworkout snack.

ROSEMARY-RUBBED SWEET POTATOES

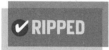

INGREDIENTS:

4	medium sweet potatoes, halved lengthwise
2	teaspoons extra-virgin olive oil
4	sprigs fresh rosemary
	Ground black pepper

HOW TO MAKE IT:

STEP 1 Preheat the oven to 400°F. Place the sweet potatoes skin side down on the oven rack. Bake for 15 minutes.

STEP 2 Refrigerate the potatoes until cool to the touch.

STEP 3 Coat a grill rack with cooking spray. Preheat the grill to medium-low. Brush each potato with a small amount of the olive oil. Pull apart the rosemary sprigs with your fingers and rub the needles onto the potatoes. Add the pepper (to taste).

STEP 4 Place the potatoes cut side down on the grill rack. Cook for 15 minutes. Flip. Cook for 10 minutes longer, or until tender.

Makes 8 servings

Per serving: 80 calories, 1 g protein, 16 g carbohydrates, 1 g total fat, 0 g saturated fat, 2 g fiber, 23 mg sodium

RIPPED TIP
If you're preparing this recipe in a Ripped Phase, substitute olive oil spray for the olive oil.

GRILLED SWEET POTATO ROUNDS

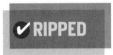 **RIPPED**

INGREDIENTS:

2	**medium sweet potatoes, sliced into ¼"-thick rounds**
1½	**teaspoons extra-virgin olive oil**
	Ground black pepper

HOW TO MAKE IT:

STEP 1 Coat a grill rack with cooking spray. Preheat the grill to medium.

STEP 2 Boil a large pot of water over high heat. Add the sweet potatoes. Cook for 6 to 8 minutes, or until tender but not soft. Drain and rinse with cold water to stop further cooking.

STEP 3 Lightly brush the potatoes with the olive oil. Sprinkle generously with the pepper (to taste).

STEP 4 Grill for 3 to 5 minutes per side, or until slightly charred.

Makes 4 servings

Per serving: 85 calories, 1 g protein, 16 g carbohydrates, 2 g total fat, 0 g saturated fat, 2 g fiber, 23 mg sodium

RIPPED TIP

If you're preparing this recipe in a Ripped Phase, substitute olive oil spray for the olive oil.

ROASTED REDS

INGREDIENTS:

4	medium red potatoes, cubed
½	teaspoon extra-virgin olive oil
	McCormick Salt Free It's a Dilly Seasoning

HOW TO MAKE IT:

STEP 1 Preheat the oven to 400°F. Coat a 12" × 9" baking dish with cooking spray. Place the potatoes in the dish. Add the olive oil. Toss to coat.

STEP 2 Sprinkle the seasoning (to taste) over the potatoes. Toss.

STEP 3 Bake for 45 minutes, shaking the dish halfway through to turn the potatoes.

Makes 4 servings

Per serving: 159 calories, 4 g protein, 34 g carbohydrates, 1 g total fat, 0 g saturated fat, 3 g fiber, 14 mg sodium

SMASHED TATERS

INGREDIENTS:

2   **pounds Yukon Gold potatoes, halved**

½   **teaspoon McCormick Salt Free All-Purpose Seasoning**

       Pinch of ground black pepper

¼   **cup fat-free milk**

1   **teaspoon chopped dried or fresh parsley**

HOW TO MAKE IT:

STEP 1   Place the potatoes in a large pot and cover with 2" of water. Bring to a boil over high heat.

STEP 2   Reduce the heat to medium. Cover. Cook for 15 to 20 minutes, or until tender through to the middle. Drain.

STEP 3   Add the seasoning and pepper. Mash with a potato masher. Add the milk a little at a time, continuing to mash until you reach your preferred consistency. If you don't use all the milk, that's fine.

STEP 4   Stir in the parsley.

Makes 6 servings

Per serving: 128 calories, 4 g protein, 27 g carbohydrates, 0 g total fat, 0 g saturated fat, 2 g fiber, 32 mg sodium

VARIATIONS: You can use small white potatoes or Idaho potatoes instead. Yukon Gold and small white potatoes don't have to be peeled, because their skins are very thin. If you're using Idaho potatoes, peel them because the skin is thicker. For an added kick, add roasted garlic to any type of spuds.

READY-MADE SPUDS

When a meal is more about function than form, I just use instant mashed potatoes instead of homemade. These take only a few minutes to prepare and make an easy side dish for any meat-and-veggie meal. All you have to do is follow the package directions. Use 100% real Idaho potatoes that come in a box or bag, and check the label to make sure they contain no fat and are low in sodium (about 20 milligrams per serving) and carbs (about 20 grams per serving).

SALADS

NO-PREP ICEBERG WEDGES

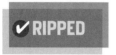 **RIPPED**

These take about 30 seconds to prep, and they look great when you plate them next to a protein-rich meal. Definitely one of my favorites.

INGREDIENTS:

1   **head iceberg lettuce**

Creamy Honey-Mustard Dressing (page 181) or any of the dressings on pages 178 to 181)

HOW TO MAKE IT:

STEP 1 Rinse the lettuce under cool water. Remove and discard any leaves that have brown spots. Cut the lettuce into quarters.

STEP 2 Serve with the dressing on the side.

Makes 4 servings

Per serving: 57 calories, 3 g protein, 13 g carbohydrates, 0.5 g total fat, 0 g saturated fat, 2 g fiber, 99 mg sodium

VARIATION: Add 8 cherry or grape tomatoes, halved.

BASIC COBB SALAD

INGREDIENTS:

1	small head iceberg lettuce, chopped
2	boneless, skinless chicken breasts, grilled and cut into cubes
2	hard-cooked eggs, chopped
2	medium tomatoes, seeded and chopped
1	avocado, cut up
1	cup grated carrots
¼	cup shredded low-fat mild Cheddar cheese

HOW TO MAKE IT:

STEP 1 Evenly divide the lettuce between two large bowls.

STEP 2 Evenly divide all the remaining ingredients between the two bowls.

Makes 2 servings

Per serving: 470 calories, 41 g protein, 24 g carbohydrates, 25 g total fat, 6 g saturated fat, 11 g fiber, 309 mg sodium

SERVING SUGGESTION: Serve with Basic Vinaigrette Dressing (page 179), Balsamic Vinaigrette Dressing (page 180), Creamy Dressing (page 180), or Creamy Honey-Mustard Dressing (page 181).

NOTE The relatively high fat content of this dish is due largely to the healthy monounsaturated fat in the avocado. Before you balk at this fatty fruit, you should be aware that it's super healthy for you. Studies show that avocados help improve serum cholesterol levels by reducing the bad stuff (LDL) and increasing the good stuff (HDL), thereby helping to protect your arteries. Avocados are also high in glutathione, a powerful antioxidant that protects cells from oxidative stress.

LOADED SPINACH SALAD

This is one of my favorites, especially when I need to replenish nutrients lost due to a hard workout. The mix of greens, vegetables, and salmon covers almost all of your nutritional bases, helping speed muscle recovery.

INGREDIENTS:

2	salmon filets (6 ounces each), rinsed and dried
1	teaspoon dried or fresh parsley
	Juice of ½ lemon
1	teaspoon + 1 pinch ground black pepper
4	cups spinach leaves
10	grape or cherry tomatoes, halved
½	cup blueberries
1	teaspoon extra-virgin olive oil
½	cup chopped sweet onion
1	clove garlic, minced
20	asparagus spears, with bottoms cut off
½	yellow bell pepper, cut into strips
1	tablespoon honey mustard (use the lowest sodium one you can find)
1	tablespoon slivered almonds

HOW TO MAKE IT:

STEP 1 Place the salmon in a deep skillet big enough for the salmon to lay flat on the bottom. Cover with 1" of water.

STEP 2 Add the parsley, lemon juice, and 1 teaspoon black pepper.

STEP 3 Bring to a boil over medium heat. Boil for 10 to 15 minutes, or until the fish is opaque.

STEP 4 Lightly scrape off the skin and fat line.

STEP 5 Evenly divide the spinach, tomato, and blueberries between two plates. Top each with half of the salmon.

STEP 6 In a nonstick skillet, combine the oil, onion, and garlic. Cook over medium-high heat for 2 minutes, or until lightly browned.

STEP 7 Add the asparagus, bell pepper, and pinch of black pepper.

STEP 8 Reduce the heat to medium. Cook for 2 to 3 minutes, or until the veggies are slightly tender.

STEP 9 Add the honey mustard. Cook for 30 seconds longer, or until the honey mustard slightly caramelizes.

STEP 10 Lay the veggies over the top of the salmon. Sprinkle with the almonds.

Makes 2 servings

Per serving: 496 calories, 42 g protein, 34 g carbohydrates, 23 g total fat, 4 g saturated fat, 10 g fiber, 237 mg sodium

NOTE Don't let the high fat content of this dish scare you. Remember, salmon is loaded with essential fatty acids—the good fat!

PEAR-WALNUT SALAD

INGREDIENTS:

¼   **cup jellied cranberry sauce**

1   **tablespoon balsamic vinegar**

½   **teaspoon extra-virgin olive oil**

     Juice of ½ orange

1   **cup mixed greens**

½   **pear, cored and thinly sliced**

1   **tablespoon chopped walnuts**

1   **tablespoon dried cranberries**

2   **tablespoons goat cheese, crumbled**

HOW TO MAKE IT:

STEP 1 In a medium microwaveable bowl, microwave the cranberry sauce on high for 20 seconds. Stir with a fork until smooth.

STEP 2 Add the balsamic vinegar. Mix.

STEP 3 Add the oil and orange juice. Mix and set aside to cool.

STEP 4 In a large bowl, combine the greens, pear, walnuts, cranberries, and cheese. Toss.

STEP 5 Serve the salad with the cranberry vinaigrette on the side.

Makes 1 serving

Per serving: 356 calories, 9 g protein, 49 g carbohydrates, 16 g total fat, 7 g saturated fat, 5 g fiber, 185 mg sodium

VARIATIONS: To make a sweeter dressing, use raspberry whole-fruit preserves instead of the cranberry sauce. To increase the protein content of this dish, add slices of Ripped Chicken (page 35).

STRAWBERRY SALAD

INGREDIENTS:

2	slices whole grain sesame bread, toasted
	Fat-free pump-spray butter
1	bag (6 to 8 ounces) mixed greens
1	pint strawberries, sliced
¼	cup chopped unsalted walnuts
1	package (14 ounces) light, extra-firm tofu, dehydrated and cubed
1	avocado, cubed
1	cup fat-free plain yogurt
2	teaspoons balsamic vinegar
1	tablespoon honey
1	teaspoon Dijon mustard
	Pinch of ground white pepper (optional)

HOW TO MAKE IT:

STEP 1 Let the toast sit for 15 minutes so it gets crunchy. Add 2 or 3 squirts of the butter spray to each slice. Let sit for 5 minutes longer. Cut into cubes.

STEP 2 In a large bowl, combine the greens, strawberries, and walnuts. Toss.

STEP 3 Add the tofu, avocado, and toast cubes to the salad. Lightly toss.

STEP 4 In a small bowl, combine the yogurt, balsamic vinegar, honey, mustard, and white pepper, if using. Mix well.

STEP 5 Serve the salad with the yogurt dressing on the side.

Makes 6 servings

Per serving: 172 calories, 9 g protein, 19 g carbohydrates, 8 g total fat, 1 g saturated fat, 4 g fiber, 161 mg sodium

SALAD DRESSINGS

Walk along the salad dressing aisle at your local grocery store, and

you'll see a ton of different ones to choose from. The problem is that

very few (if any) meet Muscle Chow standards. Just read the Nutrition

Facts labels and you'll see why. One tablespoon usually contains a lot

of sodium, unhealthy fats, and needless additives. That's why I prefer

to whip up simple salad dressings at home. Do it a couple of times,

and you'll find that it's almost as quick and easy as opening up a

bottle. Here are my five favorite recipes.

THE FORK-DRIZZLE TECHNIQUE

Awhile back, I gave my personal manager and good friend a diet plan to help him get into shape. In a relatively short period of time, he lost close to 50 pounds. He tells me all the time that friends don't recognize him anymore. His favorite part of the plan: the fork-drizzle technique. It's an easy way to shave off extra fat and calories that come standard on most restaurant salads, without sacrificing flavor.

Always order your dressing on the side. (At home, serve the dressing on the side as well.) Dip your fork (not your spoon) into the side dish of dressing and drizzle a little onto your salad. A single fork dip should last two to three bites. Repeat as you eat. Even with a huge Cobb salad (like the Basic Cobb Salad on page 173), you won't feel slighted by a lack of taste—and you'll be amazed at how much dressing is left when you're finished.

BASIC VINAIGRETTE DRESSING

INGREDIENTS:

2	tablespoons extra-virgin olive oil
2	tablespoons red wine vinegar
½	teaspoon Dijon mustard
¼	teaspoon dried thyme
¼	teaspoon minced garlic
	Pinch of ground black pepper

HOW TO MAKE IT:

STEP 1 Place all the ingredients in a bowl.

STEP 2 Mix.

Makes 2 servings

Per serving: 135 calories, 0 g protein, 2 g carbohydrates, 14 g total fat, 2 g saturated fat, 0 g fiber, 32 mg sodium

BALSAMIC VINAIGRETTE DRESSING

INGREDIENTS:

2	tablespoons extra-virgin olive oil
2	tablespoons balsamic vinegar
½	teaspoon fresh chopped basil
½	teaspoon honey mustard (use the lowest sodium one you can find)
¼	teaspoon minced garlic
	Pinch of ground black pepper

HOW TO MAKE IT:

STEP 1 Place all the ingredients in a bowl.

STEP 2 Mix.

Makes 2 servings

Per serving: 140 calories, 0 g protein, 3 g carbohydrates, 14 g total fat, 2 g saturated fat, 0 g fiber, 9 mg sodium

CREAMY DRESSING

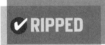
✔ RIPPED

INGREDIENTS:

¼	cup fat-free plain yogurt
1	tablespoon fat-free sour cream
1	tablespoon chopped fresh cilantro
1	teaspoon white vinegar
¼	teaspoon minced garlic
	Pinch of ground black or white pepper

HOW TO MAKE IT:

STEP 1 Place all the ingredients in a bowl.

STEP 2 Mix.

Makes 4 servings

Per serving: 11 calories, 1 g protein, 2 g carbohydrates, 0 g total fat, 0 g saturated fat, 0 g fiber, 11 mg sodium

CREAMY HONEY-MUSTARD DRESSING

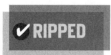

INGREDIENTS:

2	tablespoons fat-free plain yogurt
1	teaspoon spicy brown or Dijon mustard
1	teaspoon honey
1	teaspoon white vinegar

HOW TO MAKE IT:

STEP 1 Place all the ingredients in a bowl.

STEP 2 Mix.

Makes 1 serving

Per serving: 38 calories, 1 g protein, 9 g carbohydrates, 0 g total fat, 0 g saturated fat, 0 g fiber, 86 mg sodium

GREEN SALSA SALAD DRESSING

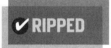

INGREDIENTS:

¼	cup Green Salsa (page 224)
1	tablespoon white vinegar
1	tablespoon Dijon mustard
1	teaspoon honey
½	teaspoon chopped dried or fresh parsley (optional)
	Pinch of ground black pepper

HOW TO MAKE IT:

STEP 1 Place all the ingredients in a bowl.

STEP 2 Mix.

Makes 2 servings

Per serving: 49 calories, 1 g protein, 10 g carbohydrates, 1 g total fat, 0 g saturated fat, 0 g fiber, 197 mg sodium

11

BISCUITS & MUFFINS

Guys who are serious about building muscle often avoid breads, biscuits, and muffins. Those foods are generally loaded with empty carbs, sugar, unhealthy fat, and, often, sodium. But there's a reason mankind has been eating bread for about as long as we've been able to walk upright: It tastes good. So don't give it up—just make it better.

I've tweaked the mix of ingredients in these baked goods to do your muscles good. Whole wheat flour fills you up with fiber and drags down the glycemic index of each recipe. Protein powder lowers the glycemic index even further, while providing the amino acids your muscles need to grow on. Fat-free ricotta cheese substitutes for butter and oil, making these muffins and biscuits moist (and adding a boost of quality whey protein). And fruits and nuts work their antioxidant magic. All in all, I think you'll find these recipes are worth the effort.

CRAN-APPLE MUSCLE MUFFINS

INGREDIENTS:

1	apple, cored, peeled, cubed, and mashed (see note)
½	cup dried cranberries
1	egg white
1	cup vanilla whey protein powder
1	cup whole grain pastry flour
1	cup fat-free ricotta cheese
3	tablespoons brown sugar
2	teaspoons Hain Pure Foods Featherweight Baking Powder

HOW TO MAKE IT:

STEP 1 Preheat the oven to 350°F. In a large bowl, combine all the ingredients. Mix well.

STEP 2 Coat a nonstick 12-cup muffin pan with cooking spray. Divide the batter evenly among the muffin cups.

STEP 3 Bake for 20 to 25 minutes, or until a wooden pick inserted into the center of a muffin comes out clean.

Makes 10 muffins

Per muffin: 158 calories, 15 g protein, 23 g carbohydrates, 1 g total fat, 0 g saturated fat, 2 g fiber, 47 mg sodium

LEAN TIP

It's easy to eat more than 1 muffin in a sitting, but limit yourself to no more than 2 per day.

NOTE It's really not tough to mash an apple with a good old-fashioned potato masher—one of the best kitchen tools you can own. I'd rather wash one masher than have to clean a food processor bowl, lid, and blade. You'll notice that none of the Muscle Chow recipes require a food processor for this very reason.

APPLE-BANANA MUSCLE MUFFINS

INGREDIENTS:

1	apple, cored, peeled, cubed, and mashed
1	banana, sliced and mashed
½	cup applesauce
¼	cup chopped walnuts
1	cup vanilla whey protein powder
1	cup whole grain pastry flour
3	tablespoons brown sugar
2	teaspoons Hain Pure Foods Featherweight Baking Powder

HOW TO MAKE IT:

STEP 1 Preheat the oven to 350°F. In a large bowl, combine all the ingredients. Mix well.

STEP 2 Coat a nonstick 12-cup muffin pan with cooking spray. Divide the batter evenly among the muffin cups.

STEP 3 Bake for 15 to 20 minutes, or until a wooden pick inserted into the center of a muffin comes out clean.

Makes 10 muffins

Per muffin: 149 calories, 11 g protein, 21 g carbohydrates, 3 g total fat, ½ g saturated fat, 2 g fiber, 18 mg sodium

LEAN TIP

It's easy to eat more than 1 muffin in a sitting, but limit yourself to no more than 2 per day.

SWEET POTATO MUSCLE MUFFINS

INGREDIENTS:

2	baked medium sweet potatoes, skins removed
2	large eggs
½	cup fat-free plain yogurt
½	cup applesauce
3	tablespoons brown sugar
1	tablespoon canola oil
½	teaspoon pure vanilla extract
1	cup unbleached or all-purpose flour
1	cup vanilla or plain whey protein powder
2	teaspoons Hain Pure Foods Featherweight Baking Powder
2	packets (2 grams) stevia or other sugar alternative
½	teaspoon ground cinnamon
½	teaspoon ground allspice

HOW TO MAKE IT:

STEP 1 Preheat the oven to 400°F. In a large bowl, combine the sweet potatoes, eggs, yogurt, applesauce, brown sugar, oil, and vanilla extract.

STEP 2 In another large bowl, combine the flour, protein powder, baking powder, stevia, cinnamon, and allspice. Add the sweet potato mixture and stir just until mixed. Don't overmix—lumps are okay.

STEP 3 Coat a nonstick 12-cup muffin pan with cooking spray. Divide the batter evenly among the muffin cups.

STEP 4 Bake for 25 to 30 minutes, or until a wooden pick inserted into the center of a muffin comes out clean.

Makes 10 muffins

Per muffin: 169 calories, 13 g protein, 23 g carbohydrates, 3 g total fat, 1 g saturated fat, 1 g fiber, 47 mg sodium

CORNBREAD

INGREDIENTS:

1¼	cups whole grain oat flour
¾	cup cornmeal
2	teaspoons Hain Pure Foods Featherweight Baking Powder
2	packets (2 grams) stevia or other sugar alternative
2	egg whites
⅓	cup + 1 tablespoon fat-free milk
1	cup fat-free ricotta cheese
2	tablespoons honey

HOW TO MAKE IT:

STEP 1 Preheat the oven to 400°F. In a large bowl, combine the flour, cornmeal, baking powder, and stevia.

STEP 2 Add the egg whites, milk, ricotta, and honey. Mix well.

STEP 3 Coat a 9" × 9" baking dish with cooking spray. Wipe away any excess spray with a paper towel. Add the batter.

STEP 4 Bake for 30 minutes, or until a wooden pick inserted in the center comes out clean.

Makes 8 servings

Per serving: 162 calories, 7 g protein, 30 g carbohydrates, 1.5 g total fat, 0 g saturated fat, 2 g fiber, 52 mg sodium

VARIATION: You can also make corn muffins by spooning the batter into muffin cups. If you do, reduce the baking time to 20 to 25 minutes.

SERVING SUGGESTION: Lightly coat your cornbread with a little fat-free pump-spray butter.

DROP BISCUITS

Every Sunday morning of my childhood, I enjoyed eating classic drop biscuits—fresh out of the oven and with a pat of butter smack-dab in the middle. Good times, but that was when I was in grade school, so they're just not part of the diet anymore. Box-mix baking products are high in sodium, saturated fat, and carbs—and they have very little to no protein or nutritional value. But those biscuits tasted so darned good that I had to find a way to get them back into my world. This recipe took me almost 20 tries before I got it right, but the end result is something I'm most proud of.

INGREDIENTS:

1	cup whole grain pastry flour
2	scoops vanilla whey protein powder
1	tablespoon brown sugar
1½	teaspoons Hain Pure Foods Featherweight Baking Powder
1	egg
1	cup fat-free ricotta cheese
1	teaspoon butter flavoring (optional)

HOW TO MAKE IT:

STEP 1 Preheat the oven to 400°F. In a large mixing bowl, combine the flour, protein powder, brown sugar, and baking powder.

STEP 2 Add the egg, ricotta, and butter flavoring (if using). Mix just until all the ingredients are incorporated. Lumps are okay, so don't overmix.

STEP 3 Coat a baking sheet with cooking spray. Wipe away any excess spray with a paper towel. Spoon out 4 biscuits onto the sheet, a few inches apart from one another.

STEP 4 Bake for 15 minutes, or until a wooden pick inserted into the center of a biscuit comes out clean.

Makes 4 big biscuits

Per biscuit: 245 calories, 20 g protein, 33 g carbohydrates, 2 g total fat, ½ g saturated fat, 3 g fiber, 101 mg sodium

SERVING SUGGESTION: Serve these straight out of the oven, nice and hot, and lightly coat with a little fat-free pump-spray butter.

PROTEIN SHAKES

12

Over the years, protein drinks have gotten more sophisticated—or complicated, depending on how you look at it. Just stroll down the protein aisle and you'll find a sea of choices, beginning with the king of all proteins, whey. Whey protein is the most popular because it tastes good, mixes easily, and is quickly absorbed and utilized by your muscles. Pick up several jugs and you'll see that each has one or a combination of a variety of whey ingredients like whey concentrate, whey isolate, whey peptides, hydrolyzed whey, ion-exchanged whey, ultra-filtered whey, and cross flow micro-filtered whey. All of which are second, third, and fourth generations of whey protein that have been broken down and filtered to help increase the biological value (BV). As I stated earlier, BV is a percentage used to determine how much protein is absorbed and retained by your muscles. Whey scores the highest of any protein source, with basic whey concentrate starting at BV 104 and whey isolates scoring as high as BV 159.

Work your way farther down the aisle and you'll find an array of casein-based proteins. Casein protein has a BV of 77, but don't let that fool you—it's not a bad thing. The reason for the lower BV score is that casein has a much slower rate of absorption (a sustained-release effect), making it a perfect protein to consume before bed. It can help you stay anabolic (in a state of muscle repair and growth) longer through the night. Casein-based proteins are also good for those times when you can't eat for several hours during the day, since they are digested more slowly and help you feel fuller longer.

Other proteins you'll see as you continue your perusal are soy, egg, vegetable, hemp, and rice proteins, for individuals who are allergic to or have difficulty digesting milk-based proteins. You'll also find low-carb proteins, weight-gainer shakes, and protein blends with nutrient additives like creatine, L-glutamine, branched-chain amino acids (BCAAs), essential fatty acids (EFAs), greens, spirulina, and a full spectrum of vitamins. Plus, there are protein products MRP and RTD. MRP stands for "meal replacement powder." This usually comes in individual-serving packets, each of which is the equivalent of an entire meal. RTD stands for "ready-to-drink." You'll most likely find these cans and bottles in the refrigerated section of health food stores. They're often consumed postworkout, in between meals, or as meal replacements.

So how do you decide which of these options is right for you? If you want a protein that you can have at any time of the day, whether in between meals, before a hard training session, or postworkout, you need a simple, fast-digesting whey protein powder that contains both whey isolates and concentrates. Because this is your "go-to" protein, get one that contains very small amounts of fat, carbs, sweeteners, or sodium. I always have at least two different flavors handy. For those mornings when you don't eat breakfast, and for pre- and postworkout supplementation, whey protein should be your first choice, since it's the fastest-absorbing protein supplement you can take.

I also use other types of protein: a casein-based protein and a weight-gainer protein. If you're going longer than three hours between meals or you want to down a protein shake before bed, a slower-digesting casein protein is best because it will keep you anabolic longer. As for the weight-gainer, it's something you might not consume every day, but it makes a great postworkout shake when you don't have time or energy for a meal.

Gainers pack around 600 calories per serving and are usually loaded with nutrients to help with muscle recovery. Check the label and you'll most likely find added L-glutamine, complex carbohydrates, some creatine, and a full spectrum of amino acids, including BCAAs. Three amino acids make up the BCAAs: leucine, isoleucine, and valine. While these are "part of the whole" when it comes to total amino acids, studies have shown that these three become depleted the most during heavy lifting and muscle exertion. In other words, all the amino acids will surely help prevent muscle breakdown while facilitating muscle repair, but BCAAs are especially important for athletes. If you're not ready to buy a gainer protein, check out the Muscle Juice recipe on page 199.

The bottom line is that shakes are the easiest way to add protein to your diet. I use the 90% Shake on page 190 about 90 percent of the time (hence the name) because it's a no-brainer to prepare and you can take it with you anywhere. While there are endless shake options, you only need a handful. Find your favorites and stick to those.

SIMPLE SHAKER-BOTTLE RECIPES

90% SHAKE

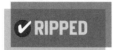

This is the shake I use 90 percent of the time because it's easy and convenient. I can travel with it anytime, anywhere. All you need is a basic shaker bottle, water, and your favorite protein powder. Premeasure single servings of the dry ingredients directly into plastic snack-sized zip-top bags so you have a week's worth of shake mixes ready to go. When it's time for a protein hit, just grab a baggie, cut off the corner, pour the mixture into a shaker bottle or regular water bottle, and shake to mix. Grab a couple pieces of fruit, and this is about as clean as it gets.

INGREDIENTS:

2	cups (16 ounces) cold water
1½	to 2 scoops protein powder (use your favorite, in any flavor)
1	tablespoon lecithin granules
1	teaspoon L-glutamine powder

HOW TO MAKE IT:

STEP 1 In a 16-ounce bottle, combine all the ingredients.

STEP 2 Shake well.

Makes 1 serving

Per serving: 216 calories, 30 g protein, 10 g carbohydrates, 4 g total fat, 1 g saturated fat, 0 g fiber, 11 mg sodium

TIP When having this shake as a late-night snack, use casein-based powdered protein instead of whey protein, to help slow the absorption process.

MALTED MUSCLES

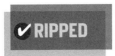

INGREDIENTS:

1	cup soy milk, fat-free milk, or water (see note)
1	cup cold water
4	tablespoons Ovaltine Malt
2	level scoops chocolate or vanilla whey protein powder
1	tablespoon lecithin granules
1	teaspoon L-glutamine powder

HOW TO MAKE IT:

STEP 1 In a 16-ounce bottle, combine all the ingredients.

STEP 2 Shake well.

Makes 1 serving

Per serving: 430 calories, 50 g protein, 36 g carbohydrates, 4 g total fat, 1 g saturated fat, 0 g fiber, 163 mg sodium

RIPPED-PHASE VARIATION: Make sure to use water rather than fat-free milk or soy milk, and reduce the amount of Ovaltine Malt to 3 table-spoons.

NOTE Soy milk will result in a thicker shake than water or fat-free milk.

NIGHTTIME ANABOLIC ELIXIR

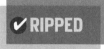 **RIPPED**

INGREDIENTS:

2	cups water
1½	to 2 scoops casein-based protein powder
1	tablespoon oat flour, or 2 tablespoons raw oats
1	tablespoon flaxseed oil
1	teaspoon L-glutamine powder

HOW TO MAKE IT:

STEP 1 In a 16-ounce bottle, combine all the ingredients.

STEP 2 Shake well.

Makes 1 serving

Per serving: 310 calories, 31 g protein, 7 g carbohydrates, 16 g total fat, 1 g saturated fat, 2 g fiber, 83 mg sodium

BLENDER RECIPES

When you use a blender to prepare your shakes, it's easy to make

them thicker and more satisfying. Just throw in a banana or, to go even

thicker, add crushed ice. You can also add a tablespoon of lecithin

granules. Lecithin, available in health food stores, is a natural

emulsifier, plus it is good for energy and helps with cholesterol and

brain function as well as vascularity.

A blender also opens up the possibility of varying your shakes with

the following ingredients:

Frozen fruit: You can add just about any kind of frozen fruit to a

protein shake. Experiment with different flavors like mango,

raspberries, peaches, blueberries, strawberries, and pineapple.

(continued)

BLENDER RECIPES (CONT.)

Nuts: Almonds provide fiber and healthy fat, plus they add texture and a light nutty flavor. Pumpkin seeds are another interesting option. A tablespoon of peanut butter or almond butter can really punch up the taste, and it goes well with a frozen banana to make a nice thick, smooth texture.

Extracts: The vanilla, almond, and peppermint extracts found in the spice aisle of any grocery store can add a bold, aromatic taste. (Peppermint is also a digestive aid that can help with flatulence; this is handy since protein shakes can sometimes cause gas.) At the health food store, you can find many other more exotic extracts: ginseng root for energy; milk thistle for liver support; silica to help strengthen hair, skin, and nails; yohimbe bark extract for energy and

sex drive; and ginkgo biloba for mental focus and circulation.

Protein additions: A tablespoon of fat-free cottage cheese or ricotta

cheese will add thickness and texture. Fat-free plain or vanilla yogurt

provides a smooth tartness. Or you can be like Rocky and add a

couple of egg whites.

A little of this, a little of that: Try a tablespoon of flaxseed oil for a

dose of omega-3s, coffee beans for a java jolt, or a tablespoon or two

of all-natural maple syrup, honey, molasses, brown sugar, or jam for

some added postworkout carbs. Add stevia for sweetness or granola

for crunch.

BREAKFAST IN A BLENDER

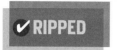

This shake is one of my morning favorites, especially when I'm heading straight to the gym for an early workout or when I don't have time to chow breakfast. The Alive! Ultra-Shake powder takes the place of your multivitamin/mineral for the day. This is one of the most complete shakes I've had—loaded with whole food vitamins, minerals, greens, herbs, amino acids, enzymes, mushrooms, and essential fatty acids. The frozen berries add taste and thickness and are packed with antioxidants. You can easily find them in ready-to-use bags in the freezer case at your grocery store.

INGREDIENTS:

1	cup frozen mixed berries
¾	cup cold water
1	scoop or 1 single-serve packet vanilla Nature's Way Alive! Rice/Pea Ultra-Shake
1	scoop protein powder (use your favorite)
1	packet (1 gram) stevia or other sugar alternative

HOW TO MAKE IT:

STEP 1 In a blender, combine the berries and water. Blend on high until smooth.

STEP 2 Add the remaining ingredients. Blend on high until fully blended.

Makes 1 serving

Per serving: 324 calories, 38 g protein, 39 g carbohydrates, 2.5 g total fat, ½ g saturated fat, 8 g fiber, 104 mg sodium

MUD PIE DELIGHT

INGREDIENTS:

1	cup crushed ice or 6–8 ice cubes
½	cup cold water
2	level scoops chocolate whey protein powder (use your favorite)
1	Weight Watchers Smart Ones Mississippi Mud Pie

HOW TO MAKE IT:

STEP 1 In a blender, combine the ice, water, and protein powder. Blend on high until mixed and frothy.

STEP 2 Add the pie. Pulse until just mixed, leaving some chunks of pie.

Makes 1 serving

Per serving: 360 calories, 51 g protein, 29 g carbohydrates, 4 g total fat, 2 g saturated fat, 1 g fiber, 86 mg sodium

CHOCOLATE ALMOND MOCHA BLAST

INGREDIENTS:

½	cup fat-free milk
1	level tablespoon instant coffee
10	unsalted almonds
1	tablespoon lecithin granules
2	packets (2 grams) stevia or other sugar alternative
1	cup crushed ice or 6–8 ice cubes
2	level scoops chocolate whey protein powder (use your favorite)

HOW TO MAKE IT:

STEP 1 Put everything except the ice and protein powder into a blender. Blend on high until fully mixed.

STEP 2 With the blender on medium, add the ice and protein powder. Blend on high until fully incorporated.

Makes 1 serving

Per serving: 393 calories, 47 g protein, 24 g carbohydrates, 10 g total fat, 1.5 g saturated fat, 2 g fiber, 55 mg sodium

MUSCLE JUICE

Packing more than 700 calories, this beast of a shake can be considered a weight-gainer that's perfect for postworkout recovery. It's also important to know that protein and carbs combined work synergistically together to make you more anabolic than just protein on its own. Here you'll find plenty of carbs to help replenish glycogen stores after a hard workout, plus added L-glutamine and creatine for muscle recovery. For the hard-gainer, this shake is all you need to put on size.

INGREDIENTS:

1½	cups fat-free milk
1	teaspoon pure vanilla extract
1	tablespoon flaxseed oil
1	teaspoon L-glutamine powder
1	teaspoon micronized creatine monohydrate (optional)
1	tablespoon natural peanut butter
¼	cup oats
1	cup crushed ice or 6–8 ice cubes
2	scoops vanilla whey protein powder (use your favorite)
1	frozen banana

HOW TO MAKE IT:

STEP 1 Put everything except the whey protein powder and banana into a blender. Blend on high until mixed.

STEP 2 With the blender on medium, add the protein powder, then the frozen banana. Blend on high until fully incorporated.

Makes 1 serving

Per serving: 769 calories, 62 g protein, 71 g carbohydrates, 26 g total fat, 3 g saturated fat, 6 g fiber, 290 mg sodium

13

SNACKS

The first Muscle Chow maneuver in dealing with a snack attack is to get rid of the old, unhealthy snacks. Go into the kitchen right now and throw out the crackers, cookies, ice cream, muffins, cereal, doughnuts, chips, pretzels, cheese, candy, etc. These muscle nemeses are especially tempting at night, when you're most vulnerable. If you don't have any of this stuff on hand, mindlessly munching on it in front of the TV won't be an issue.

The next step is to stock up on the good stuff: fat-free yogurt, no-salt cottage cheese, fresh and frozen fruit, carrot and celery sticks, raw broccoli florets, almonds, granola. And don't forget to drink water or tea to help make you feel full. Sometimes your body can confuse hunger and thirst, so try sipping instead of noshing to see if that satisfies your craving.

The key is simplicity. You just want to grab something quick. This chapter has 40 muscle-friendly options.

Part of the Muscle Chow ideal is the motto "Food with a function." Snacks are the best example of this. Sure, they defuse a raging case of the munchies, but when used correctly, snacks also serve a muscle-building purpose. There are specific times each day when you need a snack, and the following ideas will help.

PRE-PUMP FOODS

30 MINUTES BEFORE YOUR WORKOUT

A half hour before you hit the gym, it's important to consume easily digestible proteins to set the stage for optimum muscle repair and growth. A good source of protein will last you through a tough workout and beyond, until it's time to consume your next protein-rich shake or meal. As a preworkout protein boost, I like to choose one of two things: a whey-based protein shake or egg whites. Both whey protein and eggs have very high biological values (BVs), meaning they're among the protein sources most efficiently absorbed and utilized by your body.

For my favorite protein shake recipes, see Chapter 12. As far as eggs go, check out the recipes in Chapter 7. I especially like to make hard-cooked eggs ahead of time and keep them in the refrigerator for an easy grab-and-chow preworkout meal. (Check out "Hard-Cooked Eggs by the Dozen" on page 109.) You can also find hard-cooked eggs at your local grocery store in the deli or produce section, and sometimes in health food stores at the prepared foods bar. Since I chow six whites at a time, I like to keep my fridge stocked at all times with a dozen raw eggs and a dozen hard-cooked ones.

IMMEDIATELY BEFORE YOUR WORKOUT

This part is easy: A good preworkout snack is all about simplicity. Your primary focus should be on quality simple carbs for quick energy to drive you in the gym. Since you've probably already eaten a bigger meal several hours before, your glycogen stores will do the rest, offering you sustained energy to last through a grueling workout. I try to eliminate fat from this preworkout snack. Fat can interfere with vasodilation and make it difficult to achieve a pump while training. Think of this snack as a last-minute motivator to give you an extra boost, both mentally and physically, for a high-intensity workout.

Here are my standard-issue preworkout snacks—no cooking required.

LEAN PHASE

- **Snack bar.** I look for healthy, prepackaged bars that boast around 10 grams of protein, 25 grams of carbs, and 5 grams of fat—plus a little fiber to help with sustained energy. Some of my favorites include Luna Bars by Clif, South Beach Diet High Protein Cereal Bars by Kraft, GOLEAN Roll! Bars by Kashi, Zone Perfect All-Natural Nutrition Bars, and Pria Complete Nutrition Bars by Power Bar. Any of these (or anything similar) will satisfy you enough to help set the pace for a high-intensity workout.

- **Small handful of dried fruit.** Because all the water has been sucked out of them, dried fruits like raisins, apricots, figs, and dates are a concentrated powerhouse of simple carbs that offer immediate energy. They're loaded with potassium, an electrolyte that helps prevent muscle cramps and that is essential in the conversion of blood sugar to glycogen. That translates into usable energy to blast through those tough reps.

RIPPED PHASE

- **Piece of fruit.** I'll grab an apple, some red grapes, or a banana, because they offer just enough carbs to get me going (about 22 grams). Studies show that the skin and pulp of apples can help boost nitric oxide levels in the body; so can red grapes and other red-skinned fruits. (Boosting nitric oxide can lead to better a pump, which is why NO supplements have become so popular.) Bananas also contain about 400 milligrams of potassium.

- **Berries.** I store washed, cut berries in the fridge for a quick grab-and-go energy boost. Colorful fruits, especially berries, score the highest ORAC levels (oxygen radical absorption capacity), which means they're loaded with powerful antioxidants that help fight oxidative stress during a hard workout. I buy one container each of blueberries, raspberries, blackberries, and strawberries and combine them in a big bowl.

- **1 teaspoon of royal jelly.** I always keep a jar of this stuff in my cabinet for those days when I feel tired and just can't seem to get motivated to hit the gym. Royal jelly is a honeybee secretion that nourishes baby bees so they can quickly grow into large worker bees. In fact, while the life span of the average bee can be up to four months, the queen bee feeds on royal jelly exclusively and lives for up to six years.

So if this is the miracle elixir for bees, I figure it's got to be good enough to get us muscleheads off the couch and into the gym. I buy a royal jelly paste at my local health food store called Alive Bee Power by Y.S. Organics. It's a combination of royal jelly and bee pollen for stamina and energy, bee propolis for immune and anti-inflammation support, plus ginseng to help reduce stress and increase mental alertness. This is all blended in a honey base for a quick energy boost. You can find this formula (and other comparable ones) at any health food store.

- **At least 8 ounces of water.** I'll even throw in a teaspoon of L-glutamine powder to help with muscle endurance and recovery. Then I continue hydrating with water throughout my workout, especially if I'm doing cardio. It's crucial—if you're going to work up a sweat, you have to replace those fluids.

- **Greens drink.** This usually comes in powder form, but you can also find tablets, capsules, and bars. For a preworkout energy drink, I get the powder and vigorously mix it in 12 ounces of room-temperature water, then drink it about 20 minutes before my workout. It's made from plant sources like alfalfa, wheatgrass, barley grass, nuts, grains, spirulina, fruits, vegetables, seaweed, and herbal and botanical extracts. Okay, it looks like green sludge, but it has a surprisingly pleasant taste. Aside from a preworkout energy boost, a greens supplement offers antioxidant support and provides chlorophyll, which improves digestion and the body's pH balance. My favorite is GREENS Plus Wild Berry Burst by Orange Peel Enterprises.

- **Energy drink.** There are all kinds of energy drinks out there nowadays, from RTD (ready-to-drink) bottles and cans to powdered drink mixes. Most contain caffeine and stimulating herbs strong enough wake a rhino, so be careful when supplementing with any of these products. I always start with a half dose to assess my tolerance, since some of these stimulants can make you feel jittery and on edge. Just be sure to read the warning label before consuming, and seek advice from a health care practitioner if you are unaware of your current health condition or have any preexisting medical conditions.

RECOVERY FOODS

ON THE WAY HOME FROM THE GYM ...

·It's easy to overlook recovery. After all, it's something your body is doing in between workouts, athletic events, or weekend warrioring. But your recovery period is every bit as important as the amount of time you spend hoisting iron. If you train on a consistent level, it's imperative that you allow your body to fully recover, if you expect to see the best possible results.

When you work out, you're going for a pump, right? Well, achieving a pump is about creating massive blood flow into the area that you're training. Nothing feels better than hitting a muscle hard and feeling it respond by becoming bigger and more vascular than ever. Blood flow also helps shuttle out the lactic acid that you feel burning your muscles when you're hitting those final tough reps. It's also responsible for transporting oxygen to aid in faster recovery times in-between sets and exercises—the more the oxygen, the faster your recovery time.

But oxygen can also create free radicals. Heavy workouts prompt free radical production due to muscle tissue breakdown, and this can directly affect your body's ability to synthesize protein and replenish glycogen stores. Remember, working out is a catabolic process, while rest and nutrient replenishment are the anabolic polar action that ensures recovery and growth. That's why I eat the right foods—to fuel my muscles with the right nutrients for recovery, growth, and fighting free radicals.

The following recipes are my favorite postworkout meals. They can be prepared quickly so you don't waste a lot of time after a hard training session. They balance just the right amounts of muscle-building protein and glycogen-storing carbohydrates to ensure you get the most out of your hard work in the gym.

GOBBLING IS FOR TURKEYS

When you eat your postworkout meal, always concentrate on chewing well to assist proper digestion. After eating, drink a full glass of room-temperature purified water to help gastric emptying (that is, to move the protein along from your stomach to your muscles). These simple tips will ensure that you reap optimum nutritional benefits.

POSTWORKOUT EGG SALAD SANDWICH

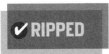

INGREDIENTS:

2	hard-cooked eggs (see "Hard-Cooked Eggs by the Dozen" on page 109)
4	hard-cooked egg whites
1	heaping tablespoon Bookbinder's Chipotle Mustard (see note)
1	teaspoon supplemental fish oil (optional)
	Dash of ground black pepper
	Dash of smoked or regular paprika
2	slices Ezekiel 4:9 Organic Sprouted 100% Whole Grain Flourless Low Sodium Bread, lightly toasted
1	box (1.5 ounces) seedless raisins

HOW TO MAKE IT:

STEP 1 In a large bowl, combine the eggs, egg whites, mustard, and fish oil (if using). Using a potato masher, mash into small pieces.

STEP 2 Add the pepper and paprika. Stir until well mixed.

STEP 3 Spoon the egg salad mixture onto one of the toast slices and top with the remaining toast slice.

STEP 4 Serve the raisins on the side to help boost glycogen-replenishing carbs.

Makes 1 serving

Per serving: 435 calories, 23 g protein, 60 g carbohydrates, 11 g total fat, 3 g saturated fat, 9 g fiber, 19 mg sodium

NOTE To locate a store near you that carries tasty Bookbinder's Chipotle Mustard, visit bookbindersfoods.com or look for a comparable brand at your grocery store. This stuff adds a low-sodium tasty kick that really makes the egg salad pop.

POSTWORKOUT ENZYME BLAST

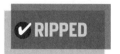

After a tough workout, you've got a two-hour window of opportunity to replenish your depleted glycogen stores in the most efficient way—with simple carbs. Therefore, it's imperative that you feed your body a quick and easily digestible meal as soon as possible. Throw some protein into the postworkout mix, and those simple carbs will also help transport tissue-repairing amino acids straight to your hungry muscles.

That's why I designed the Postworkout Enzyme Blast, because fruit is one of the most easily digested whole foods you can eat. But this isn't just any fruit; this dish is chock-full of digestive enzymes to ensure quick breakdown and assimilation that will replenish glycogen stores in a hurry—plus this recipe boasts 500 muscle-feeding calories.

☐   The pineapple and papaya are loaded with bromelain and papain, enzymes that not only help break down proteins for digestion but are also anti-inflammatory to help you heal faster and stay more anabolic.

☐   The kiwi contains protease, an enzyme that helps break down amino acids.

☐   Mango contains lactase as well as other soothing enzymes to aid in digestion. Mangos are also high in tryptophan, the amino acid that helps boost levels of serotonin in the brain, creating a sense of well-being and satisfaction.

☐   Bananas are known for their high potassium content (a great postworkout nutrient to help regulate body fluids), but they also contain amylase. This enzyme helps break down carbs into glucose, an important factor for any postworkout snack. The clove honey also contains amylase.

INGREDIENTS:

1   **kiwi, peeled and sliced**

1   **banana, sliced**

½   **mango, peeled and diced**

1   **cup fresh or canned diced pineapple**

1   **cup diced papaya**

      Juice of 1 lemon

1   **cup low-fat, no-salt cottage cheese (see note)**

1   **tablespoon clove honey**

1   **packet (1 gram) stevia or other sugar alternative (optional)**

RIPPED TIP

Reduce the carbs by using only 2 or 3 of the fruits in the ingredients list.

HOW TO MAKE IT:

STEP 1 In a large bowl, mix together the kiwi, banana, mango, pineapple, and papaya.

STEP 2 Drizzle with the lemon juice to keep the fruit fresh and prevent browning.

STEP 3 Cover and keep it in the fridge. It will last for several days.

STEP 4 When you're ready for a snack, grab a bowl and add the cottage cheese and 1 cup of the enzyme-packed fruit mix. Top with the honey.

STEP 5 If it's not sweet enough for you, add the stevia.

Makes 3 servings

Per serving: 500 calories, 48 g protein, 70 g carbohydrates, 4 g total fat, 2.5 g saturated fat, 3 g fiber, 55 mg sodium

VARIATION: Not in the mood for cottage cheese? Just put all the other ingredients in a blender, and add 2 scoops of your favorite vanilla whey protein powder, 1 cup fat-free milk, and a couple of ice cubes. Blend until smooth.

NOTE Use Friendship brand cottage cheese, if you can find it. It packs a whopping 32 grams of protein with only 100 milligrams of sodium per 1-cup serving. If Friendship is not available in your area, look for other brands that are low in sodium, like Hood, Giant, and Lucerne.

POSTWORKOUT TUNA SALAD SANDWICH

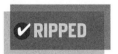 **RIPPED**

I've been prepping my tuna sandwich this way for as long as I can remember. It's clean and packed full of the perfect postworkout nutrients you need.

INGREDIENTS:

1   apple, peeled and cut into wedges

1   can (4 ounces) low-sodium chunk white tuna packed in water, drained and rinsed

1   tablespoon honey mustard (use the lowest sodium one you can find)

1   tablespoon balsamic vinegar

2   tablespoons raisins or dried cranberries

    Pinch of ground black pepper

2   slices whole grain bread

HOW TO MAKE IT:

STEP 1 Chop one of the apple wedges. Set the remaining wedges aside.

STEP 2 Put the tuna in a small bowl and break it apart with a fork. Add the honey mustard, vinegar, raisins, pepper, and chopped apple. Stir well to mix.

STEP 3 Sandwich half of the tuna salad between the bread slices. Serve with the remaining apple wedges.

STEP 4 Store the remaining tuna salad in the fridge for another postworkout meal.

Makes 2 servings

Per serving: 356 calories, 23 g protein, 60 g carbohydrates, 3 g fat, ½ g saturated fat, 8 g fiber, 85 mg sodium

TUNA IN CELERY STALKS

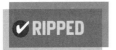
✔ RIPPED

Celery is a great postworkout food, especially if you sweat a lot during your training. It contains a balance of natural sodium and potassium, so it immediately helps restore electrolytes to your system, aiding in recovery. Of course, the benefits of chowing tuna postworkout are obvious—it provides protein to feed your hungry muscles.

INGREDIENTS:

1	**can (6 ounces) low-sodium chunk white tuna packed in water, rinsed and drained**
1	**tablespoon balsamic vinegar**
¼	**cup finely chopped onion**
¼	**cup finely chopped apple**
2	**tablespoons fat-free plain yogurt**
	Ground black pepper
14	**ribs celery, rinsed and ends trimmed**

HOW TO MAKE IT:

STEP 1 Put the tuna in a small bowl and break it apart with a fork. Add the vinegar and mix.

STEP 2 Add the onion, apple, yogurt, and pepper (to taste). Mix well.

STEP 3 Spoon an equal amount of tuna salad into the gutter of each celery rib. Arrange them on a plate, cover with plastic wrap, and refrigerate for a few hours before serving.

Makes 7 servings

Per serving: 50 calories, 7 g protein, 4 g carbohydrates, 1 g total fat, 0 g saturated fat, 2 g fiber, 80 mg sodium

RIPPED TIP

As a meal, have up to 5 servings (10 stalks).
As a snack, have up to 2 servings (4 stalks).

10-MINUTE LIME-GLAZED CHICKEN

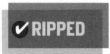

INGREDIENTS:

2   **boneless chicken cutlets**
      Lemon-pepper seasoning
      Juice of 1 lime

HOW TO MAKE IT:

STEP 1 Rinse the chicken and pat dry with a paper towel. Lightly sprinkle both sides with the lemon-pepper seasoning (to taste).

STEP 2 Coat a nonstick skillet with cooking spray. Add the chicken and cook over medium heat for 4 minutes on each side, or until no longer pink and the juices run clear. Remove to a plate.

STEP 3 Take the skillet off the heat. Add the lime juice and scrape with a spatula to create a glaze.

STEP 4 Drizzle the glaze over the chicken.

Makes 1 serving

Per serving: 260 calories, 53 g protein, 3 g carbohydrates, 3 g total fat, 1 g saturated fat, 0 g fiber, 177 mg sodium

SERVING SUGGESTION: Eat with a baked sweet potato (cooked earlier in the week; see Superhero Sweets on page 167) or a couple pieces of fruit, such as sliced mango or pineapple. Quick and easy side dishes like these will help increase glycogen-restoring carbs and make this a true postworkout recovery meal.

COTTAGE CHEESE, FRUIT & GLUTAMINE

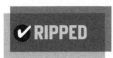

INGREDIENTS:

1½	cups low-fat, no-salt cottage cheese
1	teaspoon L-glutamine powder
1	can (16 ounces) fruit cocktail in natural juices, drained

HOW MAKE IT:

STEP 1 In a medium bowl, combine the cottage cheese and L-glutamine. Mix.

STEP 2 Add the fruit cocktail. Mix.

Makes 1 serving

Per serving: 400 calories, 44 g protein, 50 g carbohydrates, 3.5 g total fat, 2 g saturated fat, 3 g fiber, 58 mg sodium

RIPPED TIP
Substitute 1 cup fresh fruit for the fruit cocktail.

TOFU 'N' WHEY SURPRISE

Quick and easy, this stuff tastes awesome! You can make it postworkout or just about any time you feel the need for a protein kick.

INGREDIENTS:

½   package (12.3 ounces) extra-firm silken tofu (see note)

1   scoop chocolate whey protein powder (use your favorite)

HOW TO MAKE IT:

STEP 1 In a medium bowl, mash the tofu.

STEP 2 Add the protein powder. Mix until completely blended together.

Makes 1 serving

Per serving: 170 calories, 32 g protein, 7 g carbohydrates, 1 g total fat, 0 g saturated fat, 0 g fiber, 171 mg sodium

VARIATION: Double this recipe and store half in the fridge for a late-night snack.

NOTE I like Mori-Nu brand tofu because of its convenient packaging. You don't have to refrigerate it, since the airtight box prevents the tofu from being exposed to light, air, or bacteria. It stays fresh in your cupboard for a long time (see the expiration date stamped on the package). This helps maintain the integrity of the tofu, ensuring that you get the highest-quality nutrients and flavor.

VEIN-POPPIN' "TAPIOCA" PUDDING

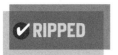

This simple snack helps replenish glycogen stores while providing a healthy dose of lecithin for cardiovascular and arterial health. Even though this dish isn't actually made with tapioca, it has a similar texture and taste. It's easy, convenient, quick, and, yes, it's made with baby food. But don't let that discourage you—the smooth pudding consistency and sweet flavor make this a tasty dessert. I suggest following it up with a basic 90% Shake (see page 190) to help boost the overall protein intake.

INGREDIENTS:

2   packages (3.5 ounces each) Gerber 2nd Foods Hawaiian Delight Dessert baby food

1   heaping tablespoon soy lecithin granules

HOW TO MAKE IT:

STEP 1 In a small bowl, combine the ingredients.

STEP 2 Mix.

Makes 1 serving

Per serving: 195 calories, 2 g protein, 40 g carbohydrates, 4 g total fat, 1 g saturated fat, 5 g fiber, 50 mg sodium

RIPPED TIP

In a Ripped Phase, only have 1 container of Hawaiian Delight Dessert and 2 heaping teaspoons of lecithin granules.

CHILI JOES

INGREDIENTS:

1	can (15 ounces) Health Valley No-Salt-Added Spicy Vegetarian Chili
4	whole wheat hamburger buns
2	cups shredded iceberg lettuce
½	cup chopped onion
¼	cup low-fat shredded Cheddar cheese

HOW TO MAKE IT:

STEP 1 In a medium saucepan over medium heat, cook the chili, stirring, for 5 minutes.

STEP 2 In the microwave, heat the buns on high for 30 seconds.

STEP 3 Evenly divide the chili among the buns.

STEP 4 Top each sandwich with equal amounts of the lettuce, onion, and cheese.

Makes 4 servings

Per serving: 223 calories, 14 g protein, 34 g carbohydrates, 4 g total fat, 1 g saturated fat, 7 g fiber, 280 mg sodium

POWER-PACKED PB&J

This promises to be the healthiest, most nutrient-packed PB&J you've ever eaten. It's a nutrient mix that makes for a perfect quick energy boost, providing a solid source of carbohydrates, usable protein, essential fatty acids, and fiber. It starts with all-natural peanut butter that you can find at your local grocery store. Don't eat this more often than once a week during a Lean Phase, though.

INGREDIENTS:

1   **tablespoon 100% whole fruit preserves**

2   **slices whole grain bread, toasted**

1   **tablespoon all-natural peanut butter**

HOW TO MAKE IT:

STEP 1 Spread the preserves on one of the toast slices.

STEP 2 Spread the peanut butter on the other toast slice.

STEP 3 Slap the two sandwich halves together.

Makes 1 serving

Per serving: 306 calories, 13 g protein, 44 g carbohydrates, 9 g total fat, 1 g saturated fat, 9 g fiber, 63 mg sodium

NOTE Don't forget to doctor up your all-natural peanut butter to make it Muscle Chow worthy. See page 33 for more details.

ON-THE-GO COTTAGE CHEESE AND PRESERVES

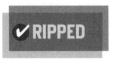

RIPPED

INGREDIENTS:

1   cup low-fat, no-salt cottage cheese

1   heaping teaspoon 100% whole fruit
     preserves

HOW TO MAKE IT:

STEP 1 In a small bowl, combine the two ingredients.

STEP 2 Mix.

Makes 1 serving

Per serving: 171 calories, 28 g protein, 8 g carbohydrates, 2 g
total fat, 1.5 g saturated fat, 0 g fiber, 30 mg sodium

VARIATION: Instead of preserves, use 1 tablespoon light maple syrup and/or 1 packet (1 gram)
stevia or other sugar alternative.

ON-THE-GO COTTAGE CHEESE 'N' BANANAS

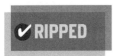
✔ RIPPED

INGREDIENTS:

1   **cup low-fat, no-salt cottage cheese**

1   **banana, sliced**

1   **packet (1 gram) stevia or other sugar alternative**

HOW MAKE IT:

STEP 1 In a small bowl, combine all the ingredients.

STEP 2 Mix well.

Makes 1 serving

Per serving: 272 calories, 29 g protein, 34 g carbohydrates, 3 g total fat, 1.5 g saturated fat, 3 g fiber, 31 mg sodium

VARIATIONS: If you don't have a banana, top the cottage cheese with a small can of well-drained fruit cocktail packed in natural juices. Or, instead of using cottage cheese, mix ½ cup soy milk with 1 scoop of your favorite whey protein powder and add the banana. Mix, cover with plastic wrap, and put it in the freezer for a rainy day.

RIPPED TIP
If you want to reduce the carbs, use only ½ banana.

ON-THE-GO YOGURT AND COTTAGE CHEESE

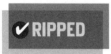
✔ RIPPED

INGREDIENTS:

1   container (8 ounces) fat-free yogurt, any flavor

1   packet (1 gram) stevia or other sugar alternative

½   cup low-fat, no-salt cottage cheese

HOW TO MAKE IT:

STEP 1 Eat half of the yogurt.

STEP 2 Add the stevia and cottage cheese to the remaining yogurt. Stir.

Makes 1 serving

Per serving: 215 calories, 22 g protein, 28 g carbohydrates, 1 g total fat, 1 g saturated fat, 0 g fiber, 130 mg sodium

PROTEIN YOGURT AND FRUIT

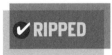 RIPPED

INGREDIENTS:

1   **container (6 ounces) fat-free plain yogurt**

1   **tablespoon vanilla whey protein powder**

1   **packet (1 gram) stevia or other sugar alternative**

       Splash pure vanilla extract

1   **cup fresh peaches, banana, or other fruit, chopped**

HOW TO MAKE IT:

STEP 1 In a medium bowl, combine the yogurt, protein powder, stevia, and vanilla. Stir until well mixed.

STEP 2 Top with the fruit.

Makes 1 serving

Per serving: 306 calories, 23 g protein, 54 g carbohydrates, 1 g total fat, 0.5 g saturated fat, 4 g fiber, 183 mg sodium

VARIATION: Add 1 teaspoon toasted wheat germ or a small handful of chopped nuts.

RIPPED TIP
Use ½ cup fruit.

CANTALOUPE WITH STRAWBERRIES AND MINT

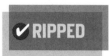
✔ RIPPED

INGREDIENTS:

½   cantaloupe, seeded and cubed

1   cup fresh strawberries, sliced

1   packet (1 gram) stevia or other sugar alternative

3   fresh mint leaves, pulled apart into pieces

HOW TO MAKE IT:

STEP 1 In a medium bowl, combine the cantaloupe and strawberries.

STEP 2 Sprinkle with the stevia.

STEP 3 Add the mint. Toss.

Makes 2 servings

Per serving: 79 calories, 2 g protein, 20 g carbohydrates, 0 g total fat, 0 g saturated fat, 3 g fiber, 26 mg sodium

VARIATION: For a slightly tangy taste, squeeze a little lemon juice over the dish.

GREEK-STYLE YOGURT

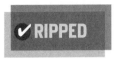

Greek yogurt is thicker and creamier than the American kind, but it can be hard to find and much higher in fat. Here's a version that you can make at home in minutes that's virtually fat-free.

INGREDIENTS:

1 **cup fat-free plain yogurt**

1 **teaspoon honey**

HOW TO MAKE IT:

STEP 1 Stack 4 paper towels on top of one another. Spoon the yogurt onto the top of the towels and spread into an even, thin layer.

STEP 2 Let sit for 1 to 2 minutes, or until the liquid from the yogurt is absorbed by the towels.

STEP 3 Scrape the yogurt into a small bowl.

STEP 4 Add the honey. Mix.

Makes 1 serving

Per serving: 128 calories, 12 g protein, 22 g carbohydrates, 0 g total fat, 0 g saturated fat, 0 g fiber, 160 mg sodium

VARIATIONS: Look closely at the ingredients lists of many flavored yogurts, and you'll likely see that they contain artificial ingredients, preservatives, and corn syrup sweeteners. Making your own flavored yogurt is easy, and you control what goes in it. These are some of my favorite mixes.

Mocha Yogurt: Mix in 1 packet (1 gram) stevia or other sweetener and ½ teaspoon instant coffee.

Cocoa Yogurt: Mix in 1 packet (1 gram) stevia or other sweetener and ½ teaspoon cocoa powder.

Berry Cream: Mix in 1 teaspoon 100% whole fruit preserves.

Maple Deluxe: Mix in 1 teaspoon all-natural or light maple syrup.

FIBER-RICH OATMEAL 'N' WHEAT BRAN

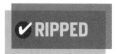

Sure, oatmeal makes a fine breakfast, but it also makes an excellent—and filling—snack anytime. I like to add bran to kick up the fiber a notch and slow the glycemic response.

INGREDIENTS:

1½   **cups water**

¾   **cup oats**

¼   **cup unprocessed wheat bran**

2   **packets (2 grams) stevia or other sugar alternative**

¼   **teaspoon McCormick Imitation Butter Flavor**

HOW TO MAKE IT:

STEP 1 In a medium microwaveable bowl, combine all the ingredients.

STEP 2 Microwave on high power for 3½ minutes.

STEP 3 Mix.

Makes 1 serving

Per serving: 298 calories, 11 g protein, 57 g carbohydrates, 4 g total fat, 1 g saturated fat, 13 g fiber, 11 mg sodium

VARIATION: If this is thicker than you like, add a little water, fat-free milk, or soy milk to thin it out.

RIPPED PHASE SERVING SUGGESTION: Serve a basic whey shake mixed with water to help increase the protein content of this meal. You can use the 90% Shake on page 190 if you'd like.

METABOLIC SALSA

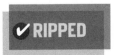

There's nothing like fresh salsa. Research shows that hot peppers actually help boost your body's metabolic rate and sustain it for several hours. A higher metabolic rate means more calories burned; more calories burned means greater fat loss. Not a bad way to spend the day on the couch watching football.

What separates this recipe from all other salsas is that it's sodium-free. If you choose to use mango, the fruit will add just enough sweetness to balance the spices and will have everyone asking, "What is that?"

If you happen to have a food processor, go ahead and use it to easily chop up all these fresh ingredients. Don't process the veggies into a puree. Just pulse them a few times to chop them into small pieces. Or make your salsa like I do—using a cutting board, a knife, and a lot of patience.

INGREDIENTS:

6	medium vine-ripened tomatoes, chopped
4	ribs celery, chopped
4	jalapeño chile peppers, finely chopped
4	serrano or other chile peppers, finely chopped (see note)
1	bunch cilantro, finely chopped
½	yellow bell pepper, seeded and chopped
1	cup chopped mango (optional)
½	cup sweet onion, chopped
½	cup key lime juice
1	tablespoon extra-virgin olive oil
	Ground black pepper to taste

HOW TO MAKE IT:

STEP 1 Put everything in a large bowl.

STEP 2 Stir to mix well.

Makes 2 quarts (8 cups)

Per cup: 54 calories, 2 g protein, 9 g carbohydrates, 2 g total fat, 0 g saturated fat, 2 g fiber, 33 mg sodium

SERVING SUGGESTION: This salsa is excellent over fish, chicken, or eggs. If you're into dipping, use baked corn chips or fresh vegetables.

NOTE Since the type of peppers available varies among grocery stores, buy whichever three or four different ones you want to use. Choose several colors to make your salsa interesting. If you want your salsa to sear, don't seed the hot peppers. The seeds contain capsaicin, the chemical that gives peppers (and your metabolism) their burn. I like my salsa so spicy that my lips are on fire, but if you prefer a milder salsa, remove the seeds.

GREEN SALSA

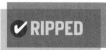

✔ RIPPED

INGREDIENTS:

2	poblano chile peppers, halved and seeded
2	serrano chile peppers, halved and seeded
1	avocado
1	clove garlic
1	bunch cilantro
½	green bell pepper, seeded and chopped
½	medium sweet onion, chopped
¼	head iceberg lettuce, chopped
½	cup water
	Juice of 2 limes
1	can (14.5 ounces) no-salt diced tomatoes, drained well

HOW TO MAKE IT:

STEP 1 In a blender, combine all the ingredients except the tomatoes. Blend until chunky smooth. (If you can't fit all the ingredients into your blender at once, add half, blend them down, then add the rest and finish blending.)

STEP 2 Pour into a large bowl.

STEP 3 Add the tomatoes. Mix.

Makes 1 quart (4 cups)

Per cup: 141 calories, 4 g protein, 17 g carbohydrates, 7.5 g total fat, 1 g saturated fat, 7 g fiber, 54 mg sodium

SERVING SUGGESTION: Use as a condiment for high-protein dishes like chicken, fish, and eggs.

TIP Because this recipe yields a lot of salsa, I like to use a little to make the Green Salsa Salad Dressing on page 181.

TANGY GARLIC DIP

This is a great condiment for raw vegetables, also known as crudités.

INGREDIENTS:

1	cup fat-free sour cream
2	tablespoons fat-free mayonnaise
	Juice of 1 lime
½	teaspoon low-salt garlic powder
	Ground black pepper to taste

HOW TO MAKE IT:

STEP 1 Put all the ingredients in a medium bowl.

STEP 2 Mix well.

Makes 18 servings

Per serving (1 tablespoon): 15 calories, 1 g protein, 3 g carbohydrates, 0 g total fat, 0 g saturated fat, 0 g fiber, 24 mg sodium

SERVING SUGGESTION: Serve the dip with baby carrots, celery, broccoli florets, cauliflower, bell pepper strips, cherry tomatoes, or cucumber—or a mix of some of each. Raw vegetables provide a great way to sit and snack to your heart's content (literally and figuratively). You'll give your body fiber, lots of phytonutrients, and rich carbs that are good for you.

BALSAMIC DIP

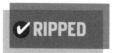

Raw broccoli is one of my favorite things to munch on while watching the tube in the evening. And I never chow a plate of it without this homemade concoction for dipping.

INGREDIENTS:

2	tablespoons balsamic vinegar
1	tablespoon honey mustard (use the lowest sodium one you can find)
½	teaspoon extra-virgin olive oil
	Pinch of ground black pepper

STEP 1 In a small bowl, combine all the ingredients.

STEP 2 Mix.

Makes 1 serving

Per serving: 70 calories, 0 g protein, 10 g carbohydrates, 2 g total fat, ½ g saturated fat, 0 g fiber, 115 mg sodium

PEANUT BUTTER MUSCLE BOMBS

These make a great on-the-go snack. Just divide the batch among zip-top bags that you can grab on your way out the door. But beware: They're dangerous—you're either eating them or thinking about eating them! To practice portion control, separate servings into zip-top bags (4 bombs per bag), store them in the freezer, and during a Lean Phase have only one bag per week.

INGREDIENTS:

2   cups all-natural unsalted crunchy peanut butter, drained of separated oil

2   scoops vanilla whey protein powder

¼   cup + 1 tablespoon molasses

2   tablespoons whole flaxseeds

HOW TO MAKE IT:

STEP 1 In a large bowl, mix together all the ingredients. This takes some muscle.

STEP 2 Form the mixture into walnut-size balls. Place in a container lined with waxed paper or parchment, separating each layer with another sheet of waxed paper or parchment.

STEP 3 Chill in the freezer or fridge for at least 2 hours before serving. (I like them best frozen, but it's your call.)

Makes 25 bombs

Per bomb: 153 calories, 6 g protein, 8 g carbohydrates, 9 g total fat, 1 g saturated fat, 1 g fiber, 46 mg sodium

MALTED ALMOND BOMBS

To practice portion control, separate servings into zip-top bags (4 bombs per bag), store them in the freezer, and during a Lean Phase have only one bag per week.

INGREDIENTS:

¼   cup Ovaltine Malt

¼   cup honey

½   cup vanilla whey protein powder

1½   cups crunchy almond butter, drained of separated oil

1   tablespoon fat-free milk

HOW TO MAKE IT:

STEP 1 In a large bowl, mix together all the ingredients. This takes some muscle.

STEP 2 Form the mixture into walnut-size balls. Place in a container lined with waxed paper or parchment, separating each layer with another sheet of waxed paper or parchment.

STEP 3 Chill in the freezer or fridge for at least 2 hours before serving. (I like them best frozen, but it's your call.)

Makes 25 bombs

Per bomb: 104 calories, 5 g protein, 6 g carbohydrates, 6 g total fat, ½ g saturated fat, 2 g fiber, 5 mg sodium

SPICY ROASTED NUTS

INGREDIENTS:

2	cups unsalted almonds
2	cups unsalted pecan halves
1	cup unsalted walnut halves
2	tablespoons extra-virgin olive oil
¼	teaspoon ground red pepper
2	teaspoons dried rosemary
2	teaspoons dried oregano
2	teaspoons smoked or regular paprika
2	teaspoons ground black pepper
½	teaspoon salt

HOW TO MAKE IT:

STEP 1 Preheat the oven to 300°F. In a bowl, combine the almonds, pecans, and walnuts. Add the oil 1 tablespoon at a time, tossing well in between to lightly coat all the nuts.

STEP 2 In a small bowl, combine the red pepper, rosemary, oregano, paprika, black pepper, and salt. Stir to mix. Slowly sprinkle the mixture over the nuts, tossing to coat.

STEP 3 Spread the nuts on a baking sheet in an even layer. Bake, stirring occasionally, for 30 to 40 minutes, or until golden brown.

STEP 4 Set aside to cool before storing in a plastic container or zip-top bags.

Makes 20 servings

Per serving (¼ cup): 240 calories, 6 g protein, 6 g carbohydrates, 24 g total fat, 2 g saturated fat, 4 g fiber, 59 mg sodium

LEAN TIP

If you're not used to practicing portion control, keeping this snack around the house can be dangerous. Snack on ¼ cup (1 serving) and no more than ½ cup up to twice a week when in a Lean Phase.

READY-MADE SNACK SOLUTIONS

The key to satisfying the munchies is simplicity. If you're like me, you just want to grab something and go. Here are a few of the things I do when I need to eat something quick.

LEAN PHASE

- **Handful of nuts.** Choose an array of unsalted nuts and seeds to create your own mixture. Dump them into a bowl, mix, and then package them individually in snack-size zip-top bags. Why go to the trouble of bagging them? Because otherwise it's too easy to sit on the couch and pound an entire bag of snack mix in one sitting. Besides, if you've got them premeasured, it's easy to grab one on your way out the door. Try to limit yourself to one bag per day.

RIPPED PHASE

- **Raw veggies.** Carrots, celery, cucumbers, broccoli, bell peppers—they're all good, especially if you store them precut in the fridge, in a container of cold water.

- **Baby food.** Seriously, I always keep a few jars on hand. It's the purest food you'll find bottled or canned. I sometimes use a fruit variety as a postworkout simple carb to replenish glycogen stores (see Vein-Poppin' "Tapioca" Pudding on page 213). Some of the vegetables are good as well.

- **Powdered protein.** No, I'm not talking about making a shake. I'm talking about taking a spoonful of protein powder right from the container to the gullet. If your protein powder is super tasty, it makes for the perfect sweet buster. You might think I'm crazy, but don't knock it till you've tried it.

- **Fat-free frozen yogurt.** Ever stand in front of the fridge wondering what you can eat that won't blow your diet? Here's a solution! Buy 6- or 8-ounce containers of fat-free yogurt (without fruit on the bottom). I like to look for interesting flavors like caramel, cappuccino, or strawberry cheesecake. When you get home, pop them into the freezer. Then whenever you want a sweet snack, microwave one for 30 to 35 seconds. It's like eating a cup of ice cream, but with more protein and calcium and less sugar. This is a great way to satisfy a sweet craving anytime.

- **Fresh or frozen fruit:** There's fruit everywhere in my house. On the counter, I keep apples, pears, peaches, nectarines, oranges, apricots, bananas, and whatever else is in season. In the fridge are cantaloupe, watermelon, berries, and grapes. There's nothing wrong with impulsively munching on any of these, so long as you're mindful of portion control (especially when in a Ripped Phase). Store-bought bags of frozen fruit

Whenever I grab a snack—whether in between meals, late at night, or any time of day—I like to keep small, 6-ounce custard dishes handy. They usually come four to a package, they're inexpensive, and you can easily find them at any grocery or department store. I have Pyrex custard cups, but 6-ounce ramekins work just as well. They're great for yogurt, cottage cheese, cut-up fruit, nuts, or any other healthy snacks you like to chow. Fill them up, and they offer just the right amount to satisfy without overdoing your portions in one sitting. They're also good when preparing recipes. You can pre-portion ingredients like chopped onion, bell pepper, or a mix of dried herbs to make it easier while cooking.

are another way to indulge a sweet craving. You can also find unique fruit blends in prepackaged smoothie mixes. While they come with healthy fresh frozen fruit, you'll also find an envelope of powdered sweetener in the bag. Do what I do—get rid of the powder and chow the fruit! Another option: Throw a bunch of grapes (on or off the vine) into the freezer and let them get rock hard. When you need a refreshing snack, these will do the trick every time.

LATE-NIGHT SNACKS

These nighttime noshes are appropriate even during a Ripped Phase.

RIPPED PHASE

- **Sugar-free or no-sugar-added frozen fruit juice bar.** A secret weapon for combatting nighttime sweet cravings; have two or three of these an hour or two before bed.
- **Fresh-brewed herbal tea.** This is a great way to end your day. I enjoy a cup or two before hitting the sack. My favorite tea for shedding excess water from between the skin and muscle is Traditional Medicinals Weightless (www.traditionalmedicinals. com). This formula contains a blend of herbs like uva ursi, bushu, cleavers, parsley, and red clover, for a gentle diuretic effect and to help suppress appetite. A cup or two at night allows me to look more ripped the next morning.
- **Low-fat cottage cheese.** Just add a 1-gram packet of stevia and mix for a great sugar-busting late-night snack. It contains glutamine to help with muscle recovery, and the protein in cottage cheese is casein-based, so it's digested slowly and helps keep you anabolic while you sleep.

14

DESSERTS

When you're building muscle, your metabolism is running overtime. Some people take that as license to splurge in their diets. If you've just burnt off an extra hundred calories with an especially grueling workout, you might think, why not take advantage of the metabolic surplus with a bigger order of fries or a decadent dessert? That mindset, my friend, separates the merely muscled from the truly ripped. Those few extra calories turn into the thin layer of fat that stands between you and a six-pack.

Now I'm not saying that you have to forgo treats—you don't. You just have to elevate their nutritional profile to make them Muscle Chow–worthy. That's what I've done with these dessert recipes. Each one trades the empty carbs you'll find in most sweets for quality carbs—the kind that give you energy while helping you feel full. Factor in some whey protein powder, low-fat dairy products, and eggs, and you have a dessert that works as hard as you do.

RASPBERRY-MOCHA CHOCOLATE CHIP COOKIES

These biceps-bustin' cookies are completely satisfying and loaded with muscle-building protein that comes from three different sources: dairy, eggs, and powdered whey. They're also chock full of cocoa powder and lecithin granules to aid in cardiovascular health and vasodilation, ensuring a better pump the next time you hit the gym. And finally, infused with coffee and a touch of raspberries, these cookies epitomize the term *healthy dessert*.

INGREDIENTS:

1½	**cups chocolate whey protein powder**
¾	**cup whole grain pastry flour**
¼	**cup cocoa powder**
¼	**cup dried raspberries**
4	**packets (4 grams) stevia or other sugar alternative**
2	**tablespoons mini semisweet chocolate chips**
2	**tablespoons instant coffee**
1	**teaspoon Hain Pure Foods Featherweight Baking Powder**
2	**eggs**
¾	**cup fat-free ricotta cheese**
½	**cup applesauce**
¼	**cup packed brown sugar**
2	**tablespoons soy lecithin granules**
1	**teaspoon pure vanilla extract**

HOW TO MAKE IT:

STEP 1 Preheat the oven to 350°F.

STEP 2 In a large bowl, combine the protein powder, pastry flour, cocoa powder, raspberries, stevia, chocolate chips, instant coffee, and baking powder. Mix well.

STEP 3 In another large bowl, combine the eggs, ricotta, applesauce, brown sugar, lecithin granules, and vanilla extract. Mix until well blended. Add to the flour mixture and mix well.

STEP 4 Coat 2 baking sheets with cooking spray. Drop the dough by spoonfuls onto the baking sheets, spaced about 2" apart.

STEP 5 Bake for 12 minutes, or until a wooden pick inserted in the center of a cookie comes out clean.

STEP 6 Remove the cookies to a wire rack to cool. When completely cooled, store in a cookie jar or container with a loose-fitting lid so excess moisture can escape.

Makes 10 cookies

Per cookie: 183 calories, 16 g protein, 22 g carbohydrates, 3 g total fat, 1 g saturated fat, 2 g fiber, 36 mg sodium

CHERRY CUSTARD PROTEIN PIE

INGREDIENTS:

4	sheets low-fat honey graham crackers, crushed into crumbs
½	cup applesauce
1	teaspoon ground cinnamon
2	cups quick-cooking oats
½	cup water
4	scoops vanilla whey protein powder
1	can (20 ounces) no-sugar-added cherry fruit filling

HOW TO MAKE IT:

STEP 1 Preheat the oven to 350°F. In a large bowl, combine the graham cracker crumbs, applesauce, cinnamon, and 1 cup of the oatmeal. Mix well.

STEP 2 Set aside 1 tablespoon of the crumb mixture. Pour the rest of the crumb mixture into a 9" × 1½" cake pan. Use the back of a spoon to press it evenly into and along the sides of the pan to form a crust.

STEP 3 In a shaker bottle, combine the water and protein powder. Shake to mix. Pour it into a large bowl and add the cherry filling and the remaining 1 cup oatmeal. Mix.

STEP 4 Pour the filling mixture over the crust. Bake for 25 minutes.

STEP 5 Sprinkle the reserved 1 tablespoon crumb mixture over the top of the pie. Raise the oven temperature to broil. Broil for 1 to 2 minutes, or just until golden brown.

STEP 6 Cool on a wire rack for at least 20 minutes before serving.

Makes 8 servings

Per serving: 208 calories, 15 g protein, 32 g carbohydrates, 2.5 g total fat, 0 g saturated fat 4, g fiber, 76 mg sodium

PROTEIN MOUSSE I

INGREDIENTS:

½	**cup cool water**
2	**scoops chocolate whey protein powder (see note)**
1	**package (14 ounces) low-fat extra-firm tofu**
1	**tablespoon chocolate syrup (optional)**
3	**egg whites**
2	**packets (2 grams) stevia or other sugar alternative**

HOW TO MAKE IT:

STEP 1 In a shaker bottle, combine the water and protein powder. Shake to mix.

STEP 2 In a blender, combine the protein shake, tofu, and chocolate syrup, if using. Blend until smooth. Transfer to a large bowl.

STEP 3 In another large bowl, whip together the egg whites and stevia until stiff peaks form. (Unless you want a serious arm workout, use an electric mixer; a whisk will take forever.)

STEP 4 Gently mix the meringue into the protein mixture.

STEP 5 Evenly divide the mousse among 4 cups or small bowls. Cover with plastic wrap. Refrigerate for at least 4 hours.

Makes 4 servings

Per serving: 105 calories, 20 g protein, 5 g carbohydrates, 1 g total fat, 0 g saturated fat, 0 g fiber, 140 mg sodium

NOTE I like to use Muscle Milk by CytoSport, American Whey double chocolate by American Sports Nutrition, Essential Protein 100% Pure Whey Powder chocolate fudge by Iron-Tek, or Lean Dessert Protein Shake chocolate fudge pudding by BSN.

PROTEIN MOUSSE II

Sometimes you just want things to be quick and easy. This version of protein mousse contains a similar amount of protein as Protein Mousse I (page 235) but takes about half the time to make. Although the texture isn't quite the same, the ease of preparation more than makes up for it.

INGREDIENTS:

2   packages (12.3 ounces each) Mori-Nu Silken Extra Firm Tofu

2   tablespoons water or fat-free milk

4   scoops chocolate protein powder (see note)

HOW TO MAKE IT:

STEP 1 Add the tofu and water or milk to a blender. Blend until smooth.

STEP 2 Slowly add the protein powder and blend until fully mixed.

STEP 3 Evenly divide the mousse among 4 cups or small bowls. Cover with plastic wrap. Refrigerate for at least 4 hours.

Makes 4 servings

Per serving: 200 calories, 33 g protein, 9 g carbohydrates, 3.5 g total fat, ½ g saturated fat, 0 g fiber, 110 mg sodium

NOTE My three favorite protein powders for this recipe are American Whey double chocolate by American Sports Nutrition, Essential Protein 100% Pure Whey Powder chocolate fudge by Iron-Tek, and Lean Dessert Protein Shake chocolate fudge pudding by BSN. If you can't find any of those, use your favorite chocolate protein powder.

MIXED-BERRY PROTEIN MOUSSE

INGREDIENTS:

1	box (3 ounces) strawberry Jell-O
1	cup boiling water
3	scoops vanilla whey protein powder
1	cup fat-free sour cream
½	pint (1 cup) fresh raspberries

HOW TO MAKE IT:

STEP 1 In a large bowl, combine the Jell-O and water. Stir until the Jell-O is dissolved. Let sit for 5 minutes.

STEP 2 Refrigerate for 10 to 15 minutes, or until it begins to set.

STEP 3 Add the protein powder. Whisk until completely mixed.

STEP 4 Add the sour cream. Whisk until frothy.

STEP 5 Fold in the raspberries.

STEP 6 Refrigerate for 4 hours or overnight, until firm.

Makes 6 servings

Per serving: 155 calories, 14 g protein, 23 g carbohydrates, 1.5 g total fat, ½ g saturated fat, 1 g fiber, 107 mg sodium

NICE ICE, BABY

When the taunting music of the Good Humor truck has you in a foul mood, turn to the frozen yogurt snacks on page 230. They're a great alternative to ice cream. Other healthy sweet treats: frozen grapes. I find these downright addictive. Be sure to wash the grapes first, then toss them in the freezer, vine and all. Frozen bananas are also awesome. Peel them and then store them in a freezer bag. They're great straight out of the deep freeze, or you can add them to a blended protein shake or smoothie. Peaches, mangoes, and strawberries are also really good frozen. Just cut them up, toss them into the freezer for a few hours, and enjoy them for an anytime snack. If you don't feel like cutting fresh fruit, check the freezer section of your grocery store for mixed fruit in bags.

PEACH COBBLER

INGREDIENTS:

3	tablespoons blueberry, raspberry, strawberry, or mixed-fruit whole-fruit preserves
1	can (15 ounces) diced peaches in water or 100% juice, drained
½	cup low-fat, no-salt cottage cheese
½	cup water
¼	cup unbleached or all-purpose flour
2	scoops vanilla whey protein powder
2	packets (2 grams) stevia or other sugar alternative
½	cup quick-cooking oats
1	tablespoon honey

HOW TO MAKE IT:

STEP 1 Preheat the oven to 350°F.

STEP 2 Pour the preserves into an 8" × 8" baking dish and spread them across the bottom. Add the peaches, spreading them into an even layer.

STEP 3 In a medium bowl, mix together the cottage cheese, water, flour, protein powder, and stevia. Pour the mixture over the peaches.

STEP 4 In a small bowl, mix together the oats and honey. Sprinkle it over the cheese mixture.

STEP 5 Bake for 30 minutes, or until bubbling.

STEP 6 Allow to cool for at least 20 minutes before serving.

Makes 6 servings

Per serving: 154 calories, 11 g protein, 25 g carbohydrates, 1 g total fat, 0 g saturated fat, 2 g fiber, 25 mg sodium

APPLE PIE

INGREDIENTS:

4   sheets low-fat honey graham crackers, crushed into crumbs

1   cup quick-cooking oats

½   cup applesauce

1   teaspoon ground cinnamon

1   can (20 ounces) no-sugar-added apple fruit filling

HOW TO MAKE IT:

STEP 1 Preheat the oven to 350°F. In a large bowl, combine the cracker crumbs, oats, applesauce, and cinnamon. Mix well.

STEP 2 Set aside 1 tablespoon of the crumb mixture. Pour the rest into a 9" × 1½" nonstick pie pan. Use the back of a spoon to press it evenly into and along the sides of the pan to form a crust.

STEP 3 Bake for 15 minutes.

STEP 4 Pour the fruit filling into the crust. Bake for 30 minutes.

STEP 5 Sprinkle the reserved 1 tablespoon crumb mixture over the top of the pie. Raise the oven temperature to broil. Broil for 1 to 2 minutes, or just until golden brown.

STEP 6 Let sit for at least 15 minutes before serving.

Makes 8 servings

Per serving: 108 calories, 2 g protein, 22 g carbohydrates, 1 g total fat, 0 g saturated fat, 3 g fiber, 60 mg sodium

VARIATION: Use cherry pie filling. It's just as good as the apple, plus it's got a nice tart kick. It's well worth making both pies if you're serving a lot of guests.

TIP Store the pie in the fridge; you can eat it chilled.

KEY LIME PIE

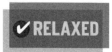

✔ RELAXED

INGREDIENTS:

4	**sheets low-fat honey graham crackers, crushed into crumbs**
1	**cup quick-cooking oats**
½	**cup applesauce**
1	**teaspoon ground cinnamon**
3	**egg yolks**
1	**can (14 ounces) fat-free condensed milk**
⅓	**cup key lime juice**
2	**cups fat-free frozen whipped topping, thawed**

HOW TO MAKE IT:

STEP 1 Preheat the oven to 350°F. In a large bowl, combine the cracker crumbs, oats, apple sauce, and cinnamon. Mix well.

STEP 2 Set aside 1 tablespoon of the crumb mixture. Pour the rest into a 9" × 1½" nonstick pie pan. Use the back of a spoon to press it evenly into and along the sides of the pan to form a crust.

STEP 3 Bake for 15 minutes.

STEP 4 In a bowl, combine the egg yolks, condensed milk, and juice. Whisk until smooth.

STEP 5 Reduce the oven temperature to 250°F. Pour the filling into the crust. Bake for 40 minutes, or until the filling is firm to the touch.

STEP 6 Let cool completely on a wire rack. Refrigerate for 4 to 6 hours, or until fully chilled.

STEP 7 Top with an even 2" layer of whipped topping. Sprinkle with the reserved 1 tablespoon crumb mixture.

Makes 8 servings

Per serving: 272 calories, 7 g protein, 53 g carbohydrates, 3 g total fat, 1 g saturated fat, 2 g fiber, 113 mg sodium

LEAN TIP

You can eat this treat during a Lean Phase if you limit yourself to just 2 servings over a 2-week period.

CUCUMBER-LIME GELATIN

INGREDIENTS:

1   package (3 ounces) lime Jell-O
1   cup boiling water
1   cup low-fat, no-salt-added cottage cheese
1   cup fat-free plain yogurt
1   cucumber, peeled and coarsely grated

HOW TO MAKE IT:

STEP 1 In a large bowl, combine the Jell-O and water. Stir until the Jell-O is dissolved. Let sit for 5 minutes.

STEP 2 Refrigerate for 10 to 15 minutes, or until it begins to set.

STEP 3 Add the cottage cheese, yogurt, and cucumber. Whisk until well mixed and slightly frothy.

STEP 4 Refrigerate for 4 hours or overnight, until firm.

Makes 6 servings

Per serving: 99 calories, 8 g protein, 17 g carbohydrates, ½ g total fat, 0 g saturated fat, 0 g fiber, 93 mg sodium

TIP You can chill this in a gelatin mold. First, lightly coat the mold with cooking spray, then wipe off the excess oil with a paper towel before adding the gelatin mixture. When the gelatin is fully set, invert it onto a plate.

MARINATED STRAWBERRIES

INGREDIENTS:

2	quarts strawberries, washed, tops cut off, and halved
	Juice of 4 lemons
1	tablespoon balsamic vinegar
1	teaspoon honey

HOW TO MAKE IT:

STEP 1 In a large bowl, combine the strawberries and lemon juice. Stir. Refrigerate for 2 hours.

STEP 2 In a small bowl, mix together the balsamic vinegar and honey.

STEP 3 Drizzle the honey vinegar over the strawberries.

Makes 4 servings

Per serving: 117 calories, 2 g protein, 29 g carbohydrates, 1 g total fat, 0 g saturated fat, 6 g fiber, 5 mg sodium

SERVING SUGGESTION: Garnish with a few lemon slices and mint leaves.

VARIATION: Instead of drizzling the honey vinegar over the strawberries, serve it on the side, for dipping.

POSTWORKOUT TIP

For a postworkout snack, chow 2 servings of Marinated Strawberries and chase them with a basic whey shake mixed with water, such as the 90% Shake on page 190.

TIP To keep strawberries—or any fruit, for that matter—from discoloring after you cut them, pour an acidic liquid like lemon juice, vinegar, or red wine over the fruit, then toss to coat.

ROASTED PEACHES

INGREDIENTS:

2	ripe peaches
¼	cup apple butter
½	teaspoon ground cinnamon

HOW TO MAKE IT:

STEP 1 Adjust the oven rack so that it's on the highest level (closest to the burners). Preheat the broiler.

STEP 2 Cut the peaches in half along the seam. Twist to separate, then discard the pit.

STEP 3 Mix the apple butter and cinnamon in a small bowl and spoon into the peach centers. Place face up on a baking sheet.

STEP 4 Broil for 5 to 8 minutes, or until browned and bubbling.

Makes 4 servings

Per serving: 67 calories, 0 g protein, 17 g carbohydrates, 0 g total fat, 0 g saturated fat, 1 g fiber, 3 mg sodium

SERVING SUGGESTION: Serve with a small dollop of fat-free frozen whipped topping, thawed.

VARIATION: Substitute apricots for peaches.

POSTWORKOUT TIP

For a postworkout snack, chow all 4 servings of Roasted Peaches, then chase them with a basic whey shake mixed with water, such as the 90% Shake on page 190.

ROASTED PEARS

INGREDIENTS:

⅓   cup apple cider

2   tablespoons brown sugar

1   tablespoon all-natural or light maple syrup

¼   teaspoon ground cinnamon

¼   teaspoon butter extract (optional)

    Pinch of ground nutmeg

3   pears, slightly underripe, peeled and halved

HOW TO MAKE IT:

STEP 1 Preheat the oven to 400°F. In a small microwaveable bowl, microwave the cider on high power for 50 seconds, or until hot.

STEP 2 Add the brown sugar and stir until dissolved.

STEP 3 Add the maple syrup, cinnamon, butter extract (if using), and nutmeg. Stir until incorporated into the liquid.

STEP 4 Use a melon baller to core the pears. Slice a small piece from the back of each pear to create a flat surface, so the fruit can lie face up in a baking dish without tipping over.

STEP 5 Lay the pears in a baking dish large enough to hold them in a single layer. Pour the cider mixture over them.

STEP 6 Bake for 35 to 40 minutes, or until the liquid bubbles and begins to caramelize.

Makes 4 servings

Per serving: 83 calories, 0 g protein, 22 g carbohydrates, 0 g total fat, 0 g saturated fat, 2 g fiber, 8 mg sodium

SERVING SUGGESTION: Top with a dollop of fat-free frozen whipped topping, thawed, or frozen vanilla yogurt.

POSTWORKOUT TIP

For a postworkout snack, chow 2 or 3 servings of Roasted Pears, then chase them with a basic whey shake mixed with water, such as the 90% Shake on page 190.

15

TROUBLESHOOTING GUIDE

Got questions? Find answers here in this quick-and-easy reference to help fix any potential problems.

MUSCLE CHOW CONCEPTS AND DIET STRATEGIES

What do you mean by "eating clean"?

When you're looking to build your best body ever, you need to fuel it in such a way that you see and feel the results of your efforts to the fullest capacity. Eating clean helps you do that, and it's what Muscle Chow is all about—more frequent, nutritionally balanced meals and snacks throughout the day; more lean proteins, fruits, vegetables, and whole grains; and fewer empty carbs. Eating shouldn't be complicated or difficult. Just make smart choices, simplify your diet, and go back to the basics: Drink more water and fewer artificially flavored drinks; eat more whole foods and fewer processed foods; and, of course, eliminate junk foods, fried foods, and fast foods.

What's a good first step to getting started with a new diet program?

First, identify the single worst thing that you're eating, then cut it by half for a week. For instance, if you're eating two slices of pizza twice a week, then have only one slice at each of those two meals. Fill in the balance with something like a salad. The following week, cut your pizza intake in half again by having a single slice just once that week. Then repeat the process with the next-worst food you're eating. After a few weeks, you'll be ready to get serious and start the Muscle Chow diet.

What foods can help reduce cravings?

Consume foods that contain both fiber and a little fat. Fiber expands in the stomach and helps you feel full, while both fiber and fat help to slow down digestion and prolong the feeling of satiety. Nuts are a good choice because they contain both fiber and fat. However, you can easily overdo it and chow too many in a single sitting, so I suggest pre-filling bags with a handful in each, to control your portions. Other fiber-fat craving busters: Protein Granola on page 56, an apple slice or celery stalk with a tablespoon of peanut butter, Avocado Breakfast on page 38, On-the-Go Cottage Cheese 'n' Bananas on page 217, or whole grain toast with flaxseed oil (see "A Toast to Muscle Growth" on page 100).

Why doesn't anything seem to satisfy me? I'm always hungry.

Sometimes the root of constant cravings is more emotional than physical. Boredom can be a big contributing factor. Also, certain routines—like watching television late at night, for instance—can be associated with raiding the cupboards. The foods you choose usually end up being something in the form of carbohydrates or sugars, and rather than satisfying you, they can make you hungrier. According to the American Heart Association, cravings may be prompted by chowing simple carbs. That's because these foods cause an insulin spike that leads to low blood sugar and stimulates hunger. Carbs also induce the release of the "feel good" hormone (serotonin) in our brains, producing a feeling of soothing calmness. When you think you're hungry and start mindlessly searching for snacks to graze on, try drinking 16 ounces of water, and you'll see how it will satisfy and calm you. If it's early in the day, I find that a cup of coffee works well. Late at night, a cup of decaffeinated tea usually does the trick.

Do you drink alcohol? If so, what do you have?

I don't drink alcohol very often, but when I do, it's usually a glass of red wine. Red wine contains healthful antioxidants, including resveratrol, a compound found in the red pigment of the grapes that has benefits such as increasing insulin sensitivity, helping maintain cardiovascular health, and improving blood flow. Of course, you can chow berries and grapes to reap these benefits, but it might not be as much fun. Alcoholic beverages also contain a form of alcohol called ethanol, which has been found to increase HDL (the good cholesterol), help prevent blood vessel damage, and control insulin sensitivity. All of these benefits are determined by one key factor—moderation. Too much alcohol (more than a glass a day) can interfere with the body's absorption of many vitamins. This includes important nutrients—like zinc, potassium, selenium, B vitamins, and magnesium—that are vital for building muscle and staying lean. Overconsumption of alcohol can also inhibit your body's ability to clear estrogen, potentially leading to side effects such as loss of muscle tone, increased body fat, and gynecomastia (male breast enlargement).

For antioxidant health, is there another alternative to red wine?

Powdered cocoa or cocoa concentrate is a viable alternative. Cocoa contains twice the antioxidants found in red wine. Be sure to check out the Raspberry-Mocha Chocolate Chip Cookies on page 233—they taste great, and the recipe calls for ¼ cup of cocoa powder. I'll sometimes add a teaspoon of cocoa powder to my morning oatmeal, along with a teaspoon of cinnamon. Cinnamon is useful because research has shown it can help control insulin sensitivity. Other options for foods with antioxidant values similar to that of red wine include blueberries, red grapes, cranberries, strawberries, raspberries, whole-fruit berry preserves, green tea, and grape juice.

Most canned and frozen foods are high in sodium. Can I eat them anyway?

Just about every section in a grocery store has low-sodium items to choose from. Some stores have tags on the shelf face (where the prices are displayed) to signify low-sodium foods. According to the FDA, the term *low sodium* printed on the package means that one serving of the food contains 140 milligrams of sodium or less. (But be sure to pay attention to the serving sizes as they can be unrealistically small.)

In the canned vegetable section, you'll always find low-sodium tomato products, peas, corn, beans, and broths. In the canned meat aisle are low-sodium tuna and sardines. Low-sodium canned chicken and salmon are more difficult to find, so be sure to drain and rinse those items before eating them, to help reduce the sodium content. As a rule, I drain and rinse these items twice (termed, double-rinsing).

The frozen section also has low-sodium foods, but they're a little more difficult to come by. The Healthy Choice brand generally contains the lowest sodium contents. If that brand isn't available, check the Nutrition Facts panel and comparison shop for sodium content.

How can I eat healthy when I'm at a restaurant?

The first option is to eat before you eat. Chow something healthy before heading out to dinner with family or friends. It can be a basic tuna sandwich (like the Postworkout Tuna Salad Sandwich on page 208), a chicken breast with veggies, or a can of salmon over a little pasta. If you don't have time, chow something easy like yogurt, a meal replacement shake, or a protein bar. This will keep you from demolishing the bread basket and will make it easy to order something light from the menu.

Once you're in the restaurant, remember you can never go wrong with a salad. Order it with plain grilled chicken or grilled fish on top and dressing on the side, then use the fork-drizzle technique (see page 178). A basic Cobb salad is always good too, so long as you order it with half the cheese, no bacon, and dressing on the side. If you're not in the mood for a salad, have a grilled chicken or grilled fish platter with plain steamed veggies. Want a sandwich? Have the same grilled chicken or fish as a sandwich; just be sure to ask for it with onion, lettuce, and tomato only.

What do you recommend eating at the movies?

Take along a bottle of water and a protein snack, such as a snack-sized protein bar containing 10 to 15 grams of protein or a meal replacement bar containing 25 to 30 grams of protein. Some of the new protein cookies are really good, or tote a bag of homemade Protein Granola (page 56). All of these snacks are easy to stash in a pocket. Even better, they'll save you 15 bucks in junk food and allow you to watch the movie with a clear conscience.

What about eating in airports?

I fly a lot and often see people devour a personal-size pan pizza in the terminal, then lumber onto the flight. Not me. I carry a meal-size protein bar like Tri-O-Plex

or Detour, throw a couple pieces of fruit in my carry-on, and purchase a bottle of water before boarding. If you forget to plan ahead, most airport shops sell Balance Bars, and fresh fruit is available in just about any airport. Here are some airport snacks I might chow.

- **Unsalted cashews or almonds.** Be careful when buying bags of nuts in the terminal because the packages usually contain much more than the recommended handful. It's a guarantee that you'll eat the entire bag if you buy it. If the shop doesn't have smaller bags, opt for the nuts you can purchase by weight and only buy a handful.
- **Balance Bars.** You can easily find these for sale in most airport shops, and they boast a decent macronutrient balance.
- **Nature Valley Granola Bars.** You can always find these in airport shops, but keep in mind that they contain very little protein and have more carbs and fat. Still, if you're in a pinch, the crunchy texture and taste will satisfy your hunger.
- **Fresh fruit, grilled chicken salads, turkey sandwiches, and fat-free yogurt.** You can find fruit by the piece at most food counters and all these other items at grab-and-go sandwich and salad shops.
- **Frozen yogurt.** There's always a frozen yogurt shop somewhere along the airport terminal to satisfy your sweet craving. Just be sure to pick a fat-free, sugar-free flavor.
- **Coffee.** Coffee can help curb your appetite and satisfy your senses, and it's guaranteed that every airport will have at least half a dozen coffee shops. Don't go for any of the blended or specialty drinks—just get coffee with artificial sweetener and a touch of cream.

BUILDING MUSCLE

I want to add more calories to my daily intake, but I don't want to eat more food.

Drink a gainer-type shake. These usually pack a whopping 600 calories per serving, they're full of complex carbs, and they boast a complete spectrum of amino acids. Some even have added muscle-building nutrients like L-glutamine and creatine. You can find these protein powders at any health food or online store that sells muscle-building products. Before you run out looking for a gainer shake, the Muscle Juice on page 199 falls into this category, boasting 769 calories per serving!

Keep in mind that you should employ this strategy only if you're serious about your training. If your workouts are sporadic or anything less than high-intensity, adding extra calories to your diet may backfire, resulting in weight gain that's not necessarily muscle.

Are there other ways to ramp up my metabolism besides eating smaller meals more often?

Another way to increase your metabolic rate is to chow spicy foods. Capsaicin, the chemical that gives chile peppers their burn, has been shown to increase metabolism for as long as five hours. Try the Metabolic Salsa on page 233. Exercise—both resistance and cardio training—plays a big role as well.

Do I need to avoid caffeine?

Caffeine has got to be one of the most popular stimulants in the world. I enjoy two cups of coffee in the morning, which yields approximately 200–250 milligrams of caffeine to help jump-start my day. Caffeine is a potent thermogenic stimulant that can increase calorie-burning potential. It can act as an appetite suppressant and helps to heighten mental clarity, and it's often used preworkout to help increase energy levels for high-intensity training. It's also been shown to help enhance endurance and blunt your threshold for pain, so you can pound out those last couple of burning reps.

Both the FDA and the American Medical Association recognize caffeine as safe when consumed in moderation. For healthy individuals, that means between 200 and 300 milligrams per day.

What foods help increase testosterone production the most?

Testosterone ranks supreme as the hormone for men when it comes to putting on lean muscle mass and maintaining a healthy libido. Foods high in protein, zinc, magnesium, saturated fat, and indole-3-carbinol not only help to optimize testosterone levels, but also play an important role in protein synthesis, prostate health, and overall well-being. Look for oysters, lean beef, lima beans, pumpkin seeds, and broccoli and other cruciferous vegetables (such as cauliflower, cabbage, and Brussels sprouts). Fats also play an important role in hormone production, so it's important to get essential fats like those found in fish, flaxseeds, eggs, and avocados.

How can I reduce estrogen levels naturally?

For men, higher estrogen means lower testosterone levels. Think of it like a seesaw between these two hormones—which can lead to a reduced sex drive, fatigue, loss of muscle mass, increased body fat, gynecomastia, and an enlarged prostate. By lowering the incidence of estrogen in your system, essentially you can increase testosterone. Chowing cruciferous vegetables may help reduce estrogen because they're high in a substance called indole-3-carbinol. In lab studies, indole-3-carbinol has been shown to reduce cells' estrogen receptors by as much as 50 percent. Some popular cruciferous veggies include broccoli, cabbage, Brussels sprouts, kale, cauliflower, arugula, collard greens, and kohlrabi. They also contain high amounts of anti-cancer phytochemicals and are high in fiber, so be sure to make some of these foods a part of your diet on a consistent basis.

You mentioned kale as a cruciferous food, but how do you prepare it?

Kale has a slightly thick, firm texture to it, so eating it raw isn't one of my favorite things to do. This is how I make it a part of my diet rotation: Start by rinsing the leaves to remove any dirt. Then cut the leaves into 2-inch pieces. Next, throw them into a pot of water and boil until the kale is perfectly tender (about 10 to 15 minutes). Drain and serve.

I'm pretty lean, but I'm still holding a little bit of thickness around my waist. How can I drop it?

Reduce your overall sodium intake; part of the weight may be water. To minimize the salt assault, Muscle Chow recipes call for low-sodium ingredients. To reduce sodium even more, cook and season with less table salt. Check the amounts of sodium in any other foods you consume and aim for less than 300 milligrams of sodium per serving.

Next, pull back slightly on your daily carbs. This will help fine-tune your body's insulin levels. Try to keep your intake below 30 grams for each snack and under 60 grams for each meal throughout the day.

Finally, be sure to hydrate with enough water throughout the day to assist in metabolic functions and to help flush your system. A realistic goal is eight 16-ounce bottles daily (or about a gallon of water).

I can't seem to lose that last little bit of water between my skin and my muscles.

Don't eat after 8:00 p.m. Before going to bed, drink a cup of herbal tea that has two or more of the following herbs in it: fennel, dandelion, uva ursi, buchu, nettle, parsley, or horsetail. These herbs have mild diuretic properties. One of my favorite teas is called Weightless by Traditional Medicinals, but there are many others to choose from, so check your local health food store. Drink a cup before bed, and you should wake up the next morning feeling slightly tighter between the skin and muscle.

Foods that have diuretic properties include asparagus, cucumbers, and watermelon. Try chowing a slice of watermelon before bed and see how you feel when you wake up in the morning. I always feel a slight bit leaner.

Can any foods help prevent muscle cramps postworkout?

If you're experiencing muscle cramps, the first thing you need to do is be sure you're hydrating with plenty of water. A gallon (or eight 16-ounce bottles) is the number you should shoot for every day. For those who sweat excessively during training, supplement with an electrolyte drink during and after your training sessions to restore lost minerals. After your workout, eat foods that are high in potassium, like baked potatoes (about 700 milligrams of potassium), a stalk of broccoli (about 500 milligrams), or a banana (about 400 milligrams). These are also good postworkout glycogen-replenishing carbs. About an hour later, have a mixed salad or a handful of raw almonds, because these are high in magnesium, a mineral that can help relax muscles. If a specific muscle is cramping, be sure to stretch and massage the area.

What does the term *afterburn* mean?

Afterburn is often used to refer to excess postexercise oxygen consumption, or EPOC, the body's ability to burn extra calories after your training session is over. How long the afterburn lasts depends on the type of training, the duration, and the intensity of your session. For instance, 20 to 30 minutes of high-intensity interval cardio training will give you a longer afterburn effect than if you do light cardio training for a longer period of time. The afterburn for resistance training is a bit different because it can last much longer than even the best cardio sessions. The reason is muscle breakdown and repair—a process that can take 48 hours or longer.

I train late at night, but then I have a hard time falling asleep. Is there something natural that I can take or do?

Try one or more of the following:

- **Make yourself a postworkout turkey, chicken, or tuna sandwich.** Each has high amounts of the amino acid tryptophan to help stimulate serotonin, the hormone that makes you feel relaxed. Just how much serotonin these foods can trigger is a matter of debate, but one thing's certain: You won't be kept awake by a rumbling stomach. Plus, you can rest easy knowing you've eaten a high-protein postworkout replenishment meal.

- **Drink a cup of chamomile tea.** Chamomile is a flower known for its calming effects.
- **Take a calcium/magnesium supplement to help relax your nervous system.** I take 500 milligrams of calcium and 250 milligrams of magnesium daily. I also chow a cup of cottage cheese before bed several times a week. Cottage cheese is high in calcium and slow-digesting protein (casein) to help keep you anabolic longer into the night.
- **Try a melatonin supplement to help promote sleep.** Melatonin, a hormone produced in the brain by the pineal gland, is mostly effective in treating sleep loss related to your circadian clock. Research suggests that melatonin decreases the time it takes to fall asleep. Pop a small dose (3 milligrams is plenty) when you need to sack out. It even comes in liquid form, so you can add it to a protein shake (such as the Nighttime Anabolic Elixir on page 192) before bed. Another option: Chow a handful of cherries. Cherries contain melatonin.
- **Look for valerian root.** It contains valerenic acid and valepotriates, two chemicals that have powerful sedative properties. A study in the *European Journal of Medical Research* found that valerian is comparable to Oxazepam, a medication sometimes used to treat insomnia. Look for the version from Nutrilite, which not only contains the most-studied formulation—450 milligrams, plus hops—but also, according to tests by Consumerlab.com, is free of contaminants.

SUPPLEMENTS

I only want to take two vitamin supplements. What should they be?

This answer can be very subjective, but here are my top two choices:

- **Multivitamin/mineral:** Taking a daily multivitamin/mineral supplement offers blanket coverage to ensure you're getting an array of nutrients you might not be getting through a balanced diet.

- **Essential fatty acids:** EFAs offer a host of benefits, like improved hormone function, joint support, healthy skin and hair, heart health, reducing inflammation in the body, and increased brain function. With well-documented benefits like these (and more), EFAs belong at the top of any supplement list.

For antioxidant health, what vitamin supplements would you suggest?

These aren't in the Muscle Chow plan, but they're certainly important vitamin supplements to consider if you want antioxidant support beyond what a multivitamin/mineral can provide. Here are my top two choices:

- **Alpha lipoic acid (ALA):** ALA is one of the most powerful antioxidant supplements you can take. The key to its potency is that it's both fat and water soluble, making it a powerful free-radical scavenger throughout all parts of the cells within your body. As if that's not enough, it also helps recycle vitamins C and E, which allows them to go much further in your system and aid in the free-radical fight. ALA can also help with cellular uptake of glucose, which is why you'll see it mixed with creatine to help with absorption—plus it increases glutathione, another powerful antioxidant that supports liver health.

- **Coenzyme Q10 (CoQ10):** CoQ10 is another biggie in the antioxidant arsenal, playing a critical role in the production of energy within every cell of your body. Benefits include heart health, immune support, and protection against free-radical damage. Be sure to look out for the newer bioactive version of CoQ10 called ubiquinol. (The regular one is called ubiquinone.) Studies are showing that it's up to eight times more powerful and effective than conventional CoQ10 (ubiquinone). For better absorption, I believe it's best to take a liquid gel-capsule rather than the dry form.

Creatine monohydrate is making me look puffy. What should I do?

Instead of creatine monohydrate, take creatine ethyl ester (CEE) instead. Creatine ester is more efficient at absorption into the muscle cell than regular monohydrate. Therefore, you don't have to consume as much product, and you don't have the water retention associated with regular monohydrate.

Is there a way I can get all the vitamins and minerals I need from food?

It's hard to beat the coverage that a high-quality multivitamin/mineral provides, but Muscle Chow can get you pretty darn close, with recipes to help you enjoy a variety of foods that are chock-full of nutrients. Also, don't forget Muscle Chow key number 5: Eat at least six servings of fruits and vegetables each day. Natural foods like these contain phytonutrients that you can't get anywhere else.

There are also multivitamin/mineral powders available (see Breakfast in a Blender on page 196).

I don't feel good when I take a multivitamin/mineral—almost feel sick. What can I do?

Here are four options to try:

1. Don't take your multivitamin/mineral on an empty stomach. After breakfast is the perfect time, but you can also take a second dose after lunch if the multivitamin/mineral you're taking requires two per day.

2. Although the bottle's serving size might be two to three tablets daily, take only one daily to get your system used to the supplement. After a week, try taking two (one post-breakfast, and one post-lunch), then see how you feel.

3. Try a different multivitamin/mineral. Sometimes your body can't assimilate a specific vitamin very well, while another won't bother you at all. Look for "whole food" type vitamins rather than synthetic ones. Often these will have a greater bioavailability than others. They tend to break up more quickly for easy digestion and absorption.

4. Instead of vitamin tablets, try different multivitamin/mineral supplement forms like veggie capsules, liquid-gel capsules, chewables, liquids, or powders.

KITCHEN TIPS

What if I don't have fresh herbs handy for a specific recipe?

You can use dried herbs, but keep in mind that they often pack a stronger punch than fresh. Because of this, use less than you would fresh—about one-fourth to one-third of the fresh amount (though measurements for parsley are the same whether you use dried or fresh).

Dried beans take so long to prepare. What's a good alternative?

Canned beans. Just be sure to look for the low-sodium or sodium-free varieties. You can find a great selection by Eden Organic—everything from adzuki to pinto beans.

How can I make my scrambled eggs and omelets fluffy?

Add a tablespoon of fat-free milk or water and use a whisk to beat the eggs for 2 minutes until they look frothy. This helps to incorporate air into the eggs, which is the key to making them fluffy. Then cook them as usual.

When cooking eggs sunny-side up in a pan, I can't see when the yolks are done.

Use a clear glass lid. This allows you to see the eggs without lifting the lid to release the steam. Just jiggle the pan back and forth a little to see if the yolks and whites are too soft. You can also tell by the color of the yolks—when they're light pink and slightly firm, they're ready. If the yolks turn yellow, you've overcooked them.

Can I cook with flaxseed oil?

No. The smoke point of flaxseed oil is low (225°F), and the oil can actually become toxic if heated too much. Flaxseed oil is best used in a finished dish—for instance, drizzled over hot drained pasta, fresh steamed veggies, rice, or salads.

Is there a good substitute for oil?

For cooking, try an equal blend of water and wine or low-sodium chicken or beef broth to help give the food some body. For sautéing, try nonstick cooking spray, then wine, water, or orange juice. When baking, use an equal amount of applesauce in place of oil.

When baking, what's a good substitute for shortening?

Fat-free ricotta cheese works well. When a recipe calls for a specific amount of shortening (or butter), I generally substitute twice that amount of ricotta. But it might take some experimenting before you find the right amount for a specific dish.

Do I need to make adjustments in cooking times for high altitude?

Higher altitudes have lower atmospheric pressure, so the boiling point of a liquid may be slightly lower. That means it can take a little longer to steam veggies or boil foods like rice and pasta, so be sure to test for doneness and make notes to gauge future cooking times. For most Muscle Chow baked goods, you shouldn't have to make any adjustments to cooking times or temperatures.

What is a leavening ingredient?

These are ingredients that help make baked dishes rise and stay fluffy so they don't fall and become as heavy as a brick. Leavening ingredients include yeast, baking soda, baking powder, and cream of tartar.

What is zest?

Zest is the outer layer of a citrus fruit. (Just the colored rind, not the white pith underneath, which can be bitter.) It's packed with essential oils, so it contains a lot of flavor. A zester works much better than a basic grater because it removes smaller bits of zest that disappear into your dish and infuse it with citrus flavor. You can find zesters at most grocery stores and all department stores.

How long does raw beef, chicken, fish, or turkey last in the fridge?

I don't like to have any raw meat sitting in the fridge longer than two days. It's best to buy what you plan to use in that time frame. After two days, throw any meat into the freezer. It'll last up to three months frozen.

How long does cooked beef, chicken, fish, or turkey last in the fridge?

I always try to consume cooked meats stored in the fridge within three to four days. After four days, it's time to toss them out.

How long do canned foods last?

I live in South Florida, so every hurricane season we stock up on canned foods. Some companies now stamp a "best by" date on their products, which helps eliminate the guesswork. Otherwise, fruits, vegetables, and soups last from two-and-a-half to three years. Canned tuna lasts up to four years, while the pouch kind stays fresh for up to three years.

ACKNOWLEDGMENTS

This is for all the people who cheered me on, supported me, and inspired me. I offer a special thank you.

To Kathy LeSage, senior editor for Rodale, who rolled up her sleeves and got in the trenches with me on this project. Her hard work and expertise helped make *Men's Health Muscle Chow* better than I ever thought it could be. For that, I thank her from the bottom of my heart.

To Phillip Rhodes, who took my ideas and concepts, simplified them, and helped make them practical and understandable.

To JoAnn Brader, manager of the Rodale Test Kitchen, for her foodstuff knowledge and thorough work on all of the *Men's Health Muscle Chow* recipe evaluations. I'm sure I drove her crazy with my many inquiries, but I also know we share the belief that success is in the details.

To Scott Quill, fitness editor for *Men's Health* magazine, who, like a good training partner, has worked with me on the "Muscle Chow" column since its inception. Thanks for the support and for always asking the right questions to spark my creativity.

To photographer Mitch Mandel for a great photo shoot. I've been around the best in the business, and Mitch is certainly one of them. Thanks for making it easy. Also, to food stylists Katrina Tekavec and M'lissa Marty, who worked closely with Mitch to bring my recipes to life and make it look effortless.

To Joanna Williams, senior book designer for Rodale, whose abundant creative talents and vision are truly inspiring. Thanks for making the cover shoot a fun collaborative effort—the end results showed.

To David Zinczenko, the savvy editor in chief of *Men's Health*, for his support throughout all of my amazing years with the magazine.

Also to: Leah Flickinger, Peter Moore, Mark Haddad, Marc Sirinsky, George Karabotsos, Hope Clarke, Marina Padakis, Faith Hague, Kayla MiChele, Mary Anderson, Nelson Scott, Billy Beck III, and Mark Pfefferman for their help and support.

And finally, a heartfelt thanks to my friends and family, to whom I owe a dept of gratitude for their limitless love and support.

To my wife, Tracy, who endured hundreds of kitchen messes, tasted my recipes, and believed in and cheered for me all the while.

And finally, to my amazing kids, Kevin and Tess, who make being a dad the greatest gift of all.

INDEX

Underscored page references indicate boxed text.

Eggs *(cont.)*
    omelets, tips for, 256
    Postworkout Egg Salad Sandwich, 205
    protein in, 97
    scrambled, tips for, 256
    separating yolks from whites, 98
    sodium in, 97
    Spanish Egg Scramble, 102
    Spicy Eggs 'n' Oats Scramble, 107
    Veggie Pancakes, 159
Energy drinks, 203
Essential fatty acids (EFAs), 19, 111, 254
Estrogen, 31, 132, 251
Extracts, adding to protein shakes, 194

F

Fats, dietary
    avoiding, in preworkout snacks, 201
    in beef, 57–58
    role in building muscle, 6–7
Fatty acids, 19–20, 111, 254
Fiber
    food sources of, 154, 246
    for reducing cravings, 246
    in apples and broccoli, 10–11
    in bulgur wheat, 34
    insoluble, about, 10
    recommended daily intake, 154
    soluble, about, 10
Fish
    Almond-Crusted Tilapia, 116
    Bamboo-Steamed Fish and Veggies, 115
    buying, 111
    canned, rinsing, 74
    canned, shelf life, 257
    checking for doneness, 112
    cooked, storing, 257
    cooking times, 111
    Easy Roasted Salmon, 114
    Fix 'n' Eat Sardine Sandy, 117
    Foolproof Grilled Fish Packets, 124
    Grilled Ahi Tuna and Vegetables, 122
    Grilled Salmon Bulgur Packets, 125
    Grilled Tuna with Peanut Sauce, 123
    Loaded Spinach Salad, 174–75
    Mahi Fish Wraps, 128
    nutritional profile, 111

    Poached Salmon with Steamed Veggies, 113
    Postworkout Tuna Salad Sandwich, 208
    protein in, 111
    Quick-Bake Fish, 112
    raw, storing, 257
    salmon, removing skin from, 114
    Sweet Tuna Salad in Romaine Boats, 118
    Swordfish on the Grill, 121
    The Fastest Rice and Veggie Dish Ever, 146–47
    Tuna in Celery Sticks, 209
Fish oil supplements, 20
Flaxseeds
    in peanut butter, 33
    storing, 30, 34
Flaxseed oil, about, 256
Food journals, 14–15
Food storage, 257
Free radicals, 18, 57, 204
Fruit. *See also specific fruits*
    adding to protein shakes, 193
    Basic Granola Energy Mix, 55
    canned, shelf life, 257
    Cottage Cheese, Fruit & Glutamine, 211
    daily servings of, 9–11
    for preworkout snack, 13, 202
    for snacks, 13, 202, 230–31, 237
    frozen, for snacks, 237
    fruit juice bars, for snacks, 231
    fruit juices, 10
    Postworkout Enzyme Blast, 206–7
    Protein Granola, 56
    Protein Yogurt and Fruit, 219
    zest, about, 257

G

Garlic
    Tangy Garlic Dip, 225
Gelatin
    Cucumber-Lime Gelatin, 241
Glucose, 7
Glutamine, 19
Glutathione, in avocados, 173
Glycemic index (GI), 8–9
Glycogen, 129, 130

Time	Food(s)	Protein	Carbs	Calories (Optional)
Totals:				